NUTRACEUTICALS

MARCEL DEKKER, INC. NEW YORK • BASEL • HONG KONG

NUTRACEUTICALS

Developing, Claiming, and Marketing Medical Foods

edited by

STEPHEN L. DeFELICE

MARCEL DEKKER

MARCEL DEKKER, INC. NEW YORK • BASEL • HONG KONG

The contents of this volume were originally published as a special issue of the journal Clinical Research and Regulatory Affairs *14(1), 1997.*

ISBN: 0-8247-0107-0

The publisher offers discounts on this book when ordered in bulk quantities. For more information, write to Special Sales/Professional Marketing at the address below.

This book is printed on acid-free paper.

MARCEL DEKKER, INC.
270 Madison Avenue, New York, New York 10016
http://www.dekker.com

Current printing (last digit):
10 9 8 7 6 5 4 3 2 1

PRINTED IN THE UNITED STATES OF AMERICA

FOREWORD

Dr. Stephen L. DeFelice coined the term *nutraceuticals* to describe a promising new revolution in medicine and health in which foods, dietary supplements, and botanical remedies are beginning to play a major role in the prevention and treatment of disease.

There is little doubt that the foundation for the nutraceutical revolution has been firmly established. Dietary modification has been shown to lower both blood pressure and cholesterol; vitamin E supplementation shows promise in the prevention of cardiovascular and Alzheimer's disease and in improving immune responses; and Ginkgo biloba is reported to improve cognition and ginseng to increase feelings of well-being in diabetics. The list is impressive and continues to grow.

The category of medical foods created by Congress is extremely important since it has already begun to encourage substantial nutraceutical research. For this reason, Dr. DeFelice convened a group of experts from diverse specialties to come together to educate all of us regarding its importance. Their outstanding contributions have been compiled in this volume.

Louis Lasagna, M.D.
Sackler School of Graduate Biomedical Sciences
Tufts University
Boston, Massachusetts

PREFACE

About a decade ago, I coined the term *nutraceutical* to give a much-needed identity and legitimacy to this amorphous nomenclatural area. A nutraceutical is any substance that is a food or part of a food and provides medical or health benefits, including the prevention and/or treatment of disease. Such products may range from isolated nutrients, dietary supplements, and diets to genetically engineered designer foods, herbal products, and processed foods such as cereals, soups, and beverages. It is important to note that this definition applies to all categories of foods and parts of food. Its range extends from dietary supplements such as folic acid used for the prevention of spina bifida to foods such as chicken soup taken to lessen the discomfort of the common cold. It applies to a bioengineered designer vegetable food rich in antioxidant ingredients as well as to a stimulant functional food or pharmafood. From a regulatory point of view, the term *nutraceutical* includes both a dietary supplement as defined under the Dietary Supplement Health and Education Act (DSHEA) and a medical food as defined in the Orphan Drug Act.

Recognizing the enormous medical–health potential of natural substances in general, the Foundation for Innovation in Medicine (FIM), over 20 years ago, began its educational effort addressing not only the promise of such substances but also the urgent need to create a research-friendly environment. I believe we have been successful. Although some would disagree, the present laws in the United States are sufficiently research-friendly to encourage corporations to establish a new medical–health sector in the nutraceutical industry. In fact, it has already happened.

CLINICAL EVIDENCE: THE DRIVING FORCE OF THE NUTRACEUTICAL REVOLUTION

The nutraceutical revolution began in the early 1980s, sparked by the calcium, fiber, and fish oil phenomena when the actual or potential clinical benefits of these substances were supported by clinical studies published in distinguished medical journals and when expert physicians began to educate their colleagues and consumers about these products via the mass media. This was followed by a continuous stream of published clinical studies defining the potential benefits of a growing range of products on a rapidly expanding array of specific disease processes. Examples include the use of Ginkgo biloba to treat certain types of dementia, niacin to prevent recurrent heart attacks, pyridoxine to treat and prevent depression, vitamin A to treat measles, magnesium to treat hypertension, garlic to reduce atherosclerosis, fish oil for hypertension, cranberry juice to prevent urinary-tract infections, vitamin E to reduce the occurrence of heart attacks, and countless others. For the first time in U.S. medicine, expert and practicing physicians—convinced by the published clinical data—joined consumers in their broad belief that foods or parts of food have medical value. This marked the entry of nutraceuticals into the mainstream of clinical practice, giving rise to an increasingly urgent need to rationalize the scientific and medical development, commercial availability, and communication about these products to the primary dual audience of physicians and consumers. Nutritionists, armed with more clinical as well as preclinical data, will play an increasingly critical role in bringing about an effective physician–consumer interface.

The promise of nutraceuticals should be considered in two ways: as potential nutraceuticals and as established ones. A potential nutraceutical is one that holds a promise of a health or medical benefit. It becomes an established nutraceutical only after there are sufficient clinical data that demonstrate such a benefit. Thus, folic acid was a potential nutraceutical until sufficient clinical evidence for the prevention of neural tube defects was generated to make it an established one, and ginseng tea remains a potential nutraceutical because of a lack of sufficient clinical evidence for any indications. It is sad to note that the overwhelming majority of nutraceutical products are in the potential category, waiting to become established.

THE NEED FOR MORE CLINICAL RESEARCH

The basic ingredients of any innovative or discovery process are: a) having an idea and b) testing it. The fewer obstacles between (a) and (b), the greater the innovative potential. For example, if Einstein or da Vinci felt the urge to create, they could simply walk to the blackboard or easel to express such creativity. The innovative process in assessing a nutraceutical, however, is vastly more difficult. It involves the nutraceutical substance (the idea) and its clinical evaluation (testing it)—a very costly process. Penicillin in a test tube is undiscovered unless it is clinically tested and found medically useful. Antioxidants that protect rodents from deleterious cardiovascular situations should be recommended only for rodents until they are proven clinically effective in humans too.

Although FIM strongly supports both basic and clinical research, FIM has always maintained that a massive influx of capital is needed primarily in the clinical research arena. In this way nutraceutical discovery can be accelerated and made available to consumers. FIM has also maintained that there is a powerful claims–research connection—the lower the cost required to make a claim, the more capital industry will invest. Associated with the reduced cost, however, is the need for corporations to have the opportunity to research and develop exclusive or proprietary products.

THE CONNECTION BETWEEN EXCLUSIVE CLAIMS AND RESEARCH

With regard to exclusivity, practical experience has well established that the availability of research-based proprietary claims leads to a research-based industry, stimulates the development and availability of technological advances, and provides a basis for regulations that facilitate and ensure accurate and approved information from companies. From a purely economic standpoint, companies desire to make medical–health claims for food products because they increase sales. Since the claims at present are not proprietary, however, the vast percentage of industry spending for such products is allocated to promotion instead of to research and development. On the other hand, in the traditional pharmaceutical industry, in which exclusive claims are usually created by the patent protection available to new molecular entities, investment in research and development is robust and the total U.S. pharmaceutical research budgets exceed that of the National Institutes of Health.

Perhaps the best evidence that exclusive claims will create a research-based industry is the U.S. Orphan Drug Act, which was designed to facilitate the commercial development and availability of drugs for rare diseases. Under the orphan drug system, testing requirements (and costs) are generally reduced and exclusive claims can be made based on company-sponsored research for a period of seven years after approval—regardless of the presence or absence of patent protection. In the 17 years prior to the Orphan Drug Act, there were only 34 approvals for orphan drugs. Since the Act was approved in 1983, however, over 400 orphan drugs have been approved or are in the research and development pipeline for the treatment of over 100 diseases, making it an outstandingly successful piece of legislation in creating a new research-based health industry.

Regarding the communication of reliable information to the physician (the key player in the nutraceutical revolution) and the consumer, clinical studies conducted for orphan drugs are presented at scientific forums and published in peer-reviewed medical journals, and thus become part of the system in which data are reviewed and scrutinized within the medical scientific community. This, in addition to a formal approval structure for medical-health claims by companies, has resulted in a medical and consumer media milieu that strives for accuracy.

DIETARY SUPPLEMENT AND MEDICAL FOODS: OPPORTUNITIES FOR DISCOVERY

And now the good news for nutraceutical research: There is plenty of room to obtain proprietary products and exclusive claims for both dietary supplements under DSHEA and medical foods under the Orphan Drug Act. Also, the costs to conduct the necessary research and development as well as marketing of nutraceutical products is quite low—from $5 million to $10 million. The time to market is approximately two years, and the profit margins can be quite healthy, well within the range of pharmaceuticals.

Companies have now begun to understand this unique opportunity to develop profitable products that will have a major impact on many discoveries within a short period of time.

THE MARKET SIZE: A DRIVING FORCE FOR RESEARCH

In terms of market size, the total U.S. retail food market in 1992 (about midway through the nutraceutical revolution) was $503 billion. This market far exceeded the combined U.S. pharmaceutical (approximately $70 billion) and OTC (approximately $24 billion) 1992 retail markets, which totaled $94 billion. It is not unreasonable to assume that 50% of that food market included foods that are used for nutraceutical reasons by consumers. It is generally accepted that dietary supplements, sugar and fat substitutes, fiber-enriched foods, vegetables, virtually fatless meat, skim milk, low-calorie diets, etc., are consumed for health or medical reasons. Coupled with the fact that 100 million Americans take dietary supplements daily, it then becomes compellingly evident that an enormous foundation for an established nutraceutical market already existed in 1992. Using 1992 data and assuming that at least 50% of food is used for medical or health reasons, we arrive at a $250 billion potential U.S. nutraceutical market, which was approximately 2.5 times the combined ethical pharmaceutical and OTC markets! It is not unreasonable to assume that in the EEC, with a larger population than the United States, the potential nutraceutical market based on 1992 data was at least equal to ours, which adds up to a combined market of $500 billion! The future estimated market is, of course, significantly larger.

CONCLUSION

I believe that the vastness of the potential nutraceutical market, coupled with the increased ability to make health–medical claims via the DSHEA and medical food categories, will lead to major corporate investment in research, primarily clinical, leading to major medical discoveries that will have dramatic impact on both the prevention and the treatment of disease. This new health sector will be manifested as a hybrid of the present U.S. OTC market. This book deals primarily with medical foods, the foundation of a new health industry. It is must reading not only for those in the corporate, government, and academic worlds but also for others who are supportive of the nutraceutical revolution and the immense promise contained therein.

Stephen L. DeFelice, M.D.

COMMENTARY: FDA PLAN (ANPR) FOR MEDICAL FOODS WOULD DISCOURAGE U.S. CORPORATE INVESTMENT IN CLINICAL RESEARCH

The Foundation for Innovation in Medicine (FIM) congratulates the Food and Drug Administration for its Advance Notice of Proposed Rulemaking (ANPR) dealing with the regulation of medical foods (61 FR 60661, November 29, 1996). FIM is particularly supportive of FDA's comments regarding the importance of producing quality products and encouraging clinical research. Unfortunately, there is a single item in this proposal that, if implemented, will nullify the general good of the ANPR, for it will have a major negative impact on the health of the American people. The proposal, which deals with the dramatic constriction of the definition of a medical food, will significantly discourage U.S. corporate investment in the clinical research that is essential to demonstrate reasonable efficacy and safety of individual medical food products. We must ask ourselves, "Do we want this?"

THE NUTRACEUTICAL REVOLUTION

"Nutraceuticals" is a comprehensive term which includes foods, dietary supplements, and medical foods, which have a health-medical benefit including the prevention of and/or treatment of disease. I coined and defined the term in order to give this new U.S. health sector a basis from which the federal government could enact rational laws that would encourage nutraceutical research, and particularly clinical trials.

The revolution began in 1983, when a National Institutes of Health consensus group recommended calcium for the prevention of post-menopausal osteoporosis. Within a very short period of time, the vast majority of Americans knew about this recommendation.

Historically in the United States, the health food industry was a consumer business largely based on traditional home and other remedies. In the early 1980s, the potential medical benefits of products such as calcium and fiber rose to prominence—with university-based clinical data to support claims for their benefits. Sparked by mass and medical media coverage, for the first time in modern U.S. medicine, physicians joined consumers in their broad belief that nutrients have medical value.

This marked the entry of nutraceuticals into the mainstream of clinical practice and scientific medical research. It gave rise to an increasingly urgent need to rationalize the scientific and medical development and commercial availability of these products, and factual communications about them, to a new audience of physicians and consumers. Clinical data stole center stage and continue to drive the nutraceutical revolution as exemplified by such products as folic acid and vitamin E.

THE FEDERAL GOVERNMENT RESPONSE

Because of increasing consumer belief and media interest in the enormous benefits of nutraceuticals, coupled with a continuous flow of positive clinical data supporting these benefits, understandable pressures were brought to bear on the federal government, which resulted in the enactment of two historic laws—the Nutrition Labeling and Education Act (NLEA) and the Dietary Supplement Health and Education Act (DSHEA). Though symbolically a major breakthrough in the psychology of permitting nutraceutical claims, the NLEA primarily discourages research because it grants the right to make a health-medical claim on a specific food or category of foods to all companies.

For example, let's assume that company A sponsors the research which demonstrates that its chicken soup reduces the morbidity (signs and symptoms) of the common cold. Let's also assume that the clinical data are sufficiently adequate to convince the FDA to grant the company the right to make that claim. FDA, according to NLEA, must then grant the right to make such a claim to all companies and not only the one that sponsored the research. Why then should company A sponsor the research? To support its competitor? Of course not! Company A will instead spend money on promotion, not research.

The NLEA, though a major step forward, is indeed a major deterrent to research-oriented companies. History has convincingly supported this view. NLEA has spawned few research-oriented nutraceutical companies.

After NLEA, the Congress passed DSHEA, which deals with dietary supplements. DSHEA, unlike NLEA, permits companies, without prior FDA approval, to make claims on dietary supplements regarding structure-function, mechanism of action, well-being, and classic deficiencies. DSHEA, however, prohibits claims regarding the diagnosis, treatment, litigation, cure, and prevention of disease.

FIM originally believed this major piece of legislation would have an immediate and highly positive effect on creating an academic-corporate, research-oriented nutraceutical complex such as exists in the traditional pharmaceutical and biotechnology industries. Unfortunately, the expected research surge is not yet evident. Companies inform FIM that the vagueness of DSHEA regarding the rules for making claims profoundly discourages research initiatives.

For example, if a company invested in clinical research which demonstrated that capsules containing a cranberry extract prevented the recurrence of urinary tract infections in women, it would not be able to make this claim. Instead of claiming, "Our cranberry extract prevents urinary tract infections"—which is the truth—it, under DSHEA, might be able to say, "Our cranberry extract provides dietary support for a healthy urinary tract," which is a half-truth and can be easily misleading.

The conclusion is that the more research one does, the less one can say about it, resulting not only in a corporate hesitancy to invest in research but also a deprivation of the delivery of nature's promise to all of us. (For the record, FIM does not fully agree with the corporate opinion regarding the degree of the negative impact of DSHEA on research. In time, FIM believes that companies will become comfortable with DSHEA and invest in research. But this is only FIM's opinion.)

MEDICAL FOODS

After the passage of DSHEA, companies, both large and small, turned to their legal consultants to advise them regarding the confusing rules of DSHEA concerning product claims. A significant number of them recommended that companies develop products as medical foods and not as dietary supplements. FDA prior approval is not necessary for a health claim for a medical food, and claims can be made regarding the positive nutritional properties of a product related to a disease, provided that corporations stress that the products must be given to patients under medical supervision.

Corporations feel much more comfortable with these clear rules for making claims. As a result, though not yet quantified, companies have initiated a substantial number of clinical studies in order to demonstrate the safety and efficacy of many medical food products.

It appears, therefore, that the medical food category has led to what we all want—an increase in preclinical and particularly clinical research. This phenomenon should not be tampered with but encouraged. It naturally follows that the degree of restriction of the definition of a medical food will be followed by a proportional decrease in clinical research. Once more, "Do we want this?"

EPISTEMOLOGIC CHAOS

After the NIH consensus group on calcium and osteoporosis, FIM predicted that future positive clinical trials of nutraceutical products would result in new federal laws that would diminish the restrictions on making health-medical claims. Because of the complexity of the situation, FIM also predicted that these initial new laws would be substantially imperfect and would periodically be improved upon as the societal nutraceutical learning curve increased. The greatest obstacle to bringing about rational changes in new laws and regulations is the attempt by the government to distinguish a health versus a medical claim.

The distinction is epistemologically false. In a vast majority of cases, there is no distinction between a health and medical claim. Both primarily deal with the prevention and treatment of disease. People consume fiber to both prevent and treat heart disease, feverfew to prevent migraine, and echinacea and chicken soup to treat the common cold—all medical indications related to disease.

Logical and effective legislation which encourages research cannot be brought about until the distinction between health and medical claims is abolished. The lack of a surge of clinical research after the passage of DSHEA is a powerful testimony to support this argument, for the health-related claims permitted in DSHEA are really medical or disease claims, yet companies are prohibited from making such medical or disease claims.

The ANPR distinguishes foods for special dietary use from medical foods. This unnecessary distinction is another example of the epistemologic chaos that creates confusion for research-oriented companies. Also, any attempt to define what constitutes a "distinctive nutritional requirement" is truly a difficult one. I would strongly recommend that a group of medical and scientific experts be assembled by the FDA to attempt to clearly define this term, for its definition will heavily affect the degree of nutraceutical research.

The principles that should determine the acceptability of claims for medical foods are qualitatively similar to those governing medical-health claims for drugs—sufficient evidence for efficacy and safety regardless of its formulation or mechanism of action.

At the 1996 FIM conference entitled, "How to Develop, Make Claims On and Market Medical Foods," FIM recommended the following guidelines for standardizing health-medical claims for all nutraceuticals.

There must be sufficient clinical data to support the claim. (The studies need not be double-blind.)

Acceptable surrogate markers (instead of clinical endpoints) can be sufficient to support a claim.

Acceptable clinical data to support the product rationale are desirable but not always necessary.

All pertinent data must be published in respected medical-scientific journals. (This is the first step of the peer review process.)

Independent consensus or expert group opinion should be obtained. (This is the second step of the peer review process.)

Post-marketing surveillance. This effort should concentrate particularly, though not exclusively, on aspects of safety.

THE DEFINITION SHOULD REMAIN UNCHANGED

If our society is to enjoy the enormous benefits that ongoing medical food research would bring about, then it is imperative that the definition of the medical food remain unchanged. There is little evidence that DSHEA and the category of "foods for special dietary use" have sparked a surge of corporate preclinical and clinical research. On the other hand, it is common knowledge among industry observers that the medical food regulations have indeed sparked an abundance of research.

Considering all the aforementioned points, the wise position would be for all of us to wait a few years to determine, in a quantifiable way, the impact of DSHEA and medical foods on the availability of products with demonstrated health-medical benefits that will positively affect the prevention and treatment of disease.

FDA is particularly concerned about the increasing number of insufficiently substantiated health-medical claims being made by companies, many of which can be characterized as charlatanic. An effective way to increase such charlatanic behavior would be to constrict the definition of a medical food which, as repeatedly mentioned here, would decrease clinical research, which is necessary to support truthful claims. The generation and promotion of sound clinical data supporting effective and safe products is the best way to drive out poorly documented or bad ones.

Stephen L. DeFelice, M.D.

CONTENTS

THE NUTRACEUTICAL REVOLUTION: WHAT IS IT?

Stephen L. DeFelice, M.D.
The Foundation For Innovation in Medicine
Cranford
N.J. 07016

The Nutraceutical Revolution can be briefly categorized as follows:

1. It represents a new and legitimate era in medicine where dietary supplements and medical foods will have a major impact on the practice of medicine both in the prevention and treatment of disease.

2. The revolution is driven by credible clinical data.

3. Nutraceuticals are now commonly accepted by consumers (both the sick and the healthy), physicians, other health care professionals and the Congress.

4. A major new characteristic of the movement of the revolution is that all have the right to receive information concerning the benefits of nutraceuticals (health-medical claims).

5. A unique and historical characterisic of the revolution is that companies and not the government, can now determine the nature of the health-medical claim and proceed to educate all segments of American society.

WHAT IS THE NATURE OF THE NUTRACEUTICAL MARKET?

1. The Foundation for Innovation in Medicine (FIM) estimates the size of the U.S. market to be $250 billion - approximately three times larger than the U.S. pharmaceutical market.

2. The present market is comprised mostly of potential nutraceuticals lacking clinical evidence to support the clinical promise. With increasing clinical research, the percentage of the potential nutraceutical market will decrease and the true nutraceutical market will increase. The players involve all types of companies ranging from food, drug, to biotech and start-up companies - a new powerful market phenomenon which is not yet fully appreciated by the corporate health sector.

3. The average cost for entry into the market is approximately $10 million - one fortieth of that of a pharmaceutical.

4. The average time of entry is approximately two years - one fifth of that of a pharmaceutical product.

5. The profit margins are robust, similar to those of pharmaceuticals.

WHERE IS IT?

Many individuals and companies contact FIM regarding various types of nutraceutical ventures. FIM has become the virtual eyes and ears of the world in this area. There are many small start-up companies now embarking on the research and development of medical foods and dietary supplements. One such company is AMBI with its salt alternative, Cardia. In the giant food industry, Ocean Spray, Campbells and Kelloggs are leading the way. Baker Norton, a division of the large pharmaceutical company, IVAX, has recently launched Zbar to reduce hypoglycemia in diabetics.

In the past year there has been a powerful surge of activity in all of these sectors.

What is highly novel and revolutionary about this surge is that many products will be marketed to the same types of patients or healthy folks. For example, should a physician recommend to a hypertensive patient a food company's special diet that lowers blood pressure or a drug company's anti-hypertensive pill or a health food company's dietary supplement? Should patients already on anti-hypertensive drugs be weaned from their drugs to the food company's special diet?

There is little doubt that special formulations will dominate this market though I find little support for my strong felt position. The literature clearly states that supplementation and not diet is where the nutraceutical benefits lay. We need more calcium, folic acid, carnitine, vitamin E, magnesium, etc. and not less. Oftentimes the amounts of supplementation needed would require too many pills or tablets a day to achieve sufficient consumer compliance. To overcome this barrier, special formulations that are consumer friendly will dominate the market, particularly liquid ones.

The current surge in nutraceutical clinical research and development is targeted to the medical food and not the dietary supplement market. This has happened mainly because the groundrules for making health-medical claims with medical foods are clearer than with dietary supplements under DSHEA. I personally believe that the opportunities for dietary supplements under DSHEA are far more flexible and effective than those with medical foods. I believe that the rush for medical foods is based on an ignorance of the dynamics of the marketplace of the nutraceutical revolution.

WHERE IS IT GOING?

And finally, the clear and present distinction between the two great health industries - food and drug - will disappear. In fact, it is happening now. New types of giant hybrid corporations will appear, fed by nutraceutical products developed by small companies. Many new nutraceutical companies will arise. These corporations will have, though presently unrecognized, a major beneficial impact on the health of the American people far exceeding present expections which will also result in a significant decrease in health costs.

MEDICAL FOODS

Jur Strobos, M.D., Esq
Greenberg Traurig
Washington, DC

I. BACKGROUND

A. Foods for Special Dietary Use

A category of products called "foods for special dietary use" ("FSDU") was created within the Federal Food, Drug, and Cosmetic Act ("FDC Act") by enactment of the Health Research and Health Services Amendment of 1976 (known as the Proxmire Amendment). The Proxmire Amendment was designed to prevent the U.S. Food and Drug Administration ("FDA") from regulating vitamins and minerals as drugs based on form (*e.g.*, tablet, capsule, gel) or dosage strength.

FSDU are statutorily defined as:

> **a food which purports or is represented to be used, including but not limited to the following:**
>
> **(A) Supplying a special dietary need that exists by reason of a physical, physiological, pathological, or other condition, including but not limited to the condition of disease, convalescence, pregnancy, lactation, infancy, allergic hypersensitivity to food, underweight, overweight, or the need to control the intake of sodium.**
>
> **(B) Supplying a vitamin, mineral, or other ingredient for use by man to supplement his diet by increasing the total dietary intake.**
>
> **(C) Supplying a special dietary need by reason of being a food for use as the sole item of the diet.**

§ 411(c)(3) of the FDC Act.

While § 411 was amended by the Dietary Supplements Health and Education Act of 1994, the definition of FSDU was unchanged.

FDA has issued a number of regulations governing FSDU in Part 105 of the Code of Federal Regulations (CFR). In particular, there are regulations on hypoallergenic foods (21 C.F.R. § 105.62); infant foods (§105.65); weight reduction foods (§ 105.66); foods for diabetics (§ 105.67); and, foods for sodium restricted diets (§ 105.69). In general, however, issuance of regulations for FSDU is cumbersome because regulations issued under § 411 of the FDC Act are subject to procedural protections found § 701(e) of the FDC Act. This section limits promulgation of regulations to formal rulemaking which includes an evidentiary hearing. The difficulty of developing timely regulations has, thus, decreased the usefulness of this category of products.

B. The Orphan Drug Act of 1983

Fortuitously, a series of subsequent enactments created a potential new category of products called "medical foods." The Orphan Drug Act of 1983 provided for designation of orphan drug products by FDA, federal funding for clinical research for such products, and a period of marketing exclusivity for orphan drugs when approved. In 1988, when the orphan drug program was up for re-authorization, Congress amended the act to extend its scope in part to include orphan devices and orphan medical foods. As stated in the legislative history:

> Since the Committee's first hearing in 1980 on orphan drugs, the Committee has received testimony and inquiries about similar problems in the development of orphan medical devices and foods. The Committee has considered on several occasions the need to extend some or all of the benefits of the orphan drug law and program to medical devices and foods, but has never done so because of the significant differences in the drug, device and medical food industries, and the laws regulating them. These differences raise important questions about the applicability of the orphan drug law and program to medical devices and foods.

> The Committee is not prepared at this time to propose such a broadening of the entire law. The Committee bill does, however, expand the orphan drug grant program so that grants could be awarded for the testing of orphan medical devices and foods.
> In addition, the Committee's bill requires the Secretary of HHS to conduct a study to determine whether application of the other provisions of the orphan drug law to orphan medical devices and foods is needed in order to encourage the development of orphan medical devices and foods. The study is due within one year of the enactment of this bill. The study would, among other things, evaluate whether the incentive for orphan drugs would serve as incentives for medical devices and foods, or whether other types of incentives would be more appropriate due to differences in the development process and the economics of the marketplace for devices and foods.

H.R. No. 100-473, 100th Cong. 2nd Sess. 8 (1988).

The definition of a medical food closely parallels but is not identical to that of a FSDU. Medical foods are defined as:

> a food which is formulated to be consumed or administered enterally under the supervision of a physician and which is intended for the specific dietary management of a disease or condition for which distinctive nutritional requirements, based on recognized scientific principles, are established by medical evaluation.

Orphan Drug Act of 1983, § 5(b)(3), codified at 21 U.S.C. § 360ee(b)(3).

The question that immediately arises is whether a food that "[s]uppl[ies] a special dietary need that exists by reason of a physical, physiological, pathological, or other condition differs from one which is "intended for the specific dietary management of a disease or condition for which distinctive nutritional requirements, based on recognized scientific principles, are established by medical evaluation." In answering this question, the legislative history is not helpful. There are those who believe the differences may have been purely accidental or unintended. However, under long-standing principles of statutory construction, one may not presume or suppose that Congress provided different words to describe the same thing.

In short, whatever they are, medical foods are not foods for special dietary use. Further, regulations for medical foods need not be promulgated pursuant to formal rule-making.

C. The Nutrition Labeling and Education Act of 1990

The current statutory history of medical foods was completed with the enactment of the Nutrition Labeling and Education Act of 1990 ("NLEA"). The NLEA provided for promulgation of regulations, among others, relating to nutrient content and nutrient content claims. The NLEA accomplished this result by exempting products which met these regulations from the misbranding provisions of the FDC Act. *See* § 403(q). Regulations have been promulgated that define nutrient content labeling, permissible nutrient content claims, and authorized health claims. Similarly, the NLEA provided for authorization of specific health claims on petition for eligible foods. *See* § 403(r). However, medical foods, as defined in § 5(b)(3) of the Orphan Drug Act, were exempted from the new § 403(r).

Health claims are statements on the labeling of foods which "characterizes the relationship" of a food substance to "a disease or a health-related condition." § 403(r). Health claims are subject to prior authorization by FDA before they may be used on a food product or the product is misbranded by virtue of § 403(r) as well as the general misbranding provisions of the FDC Act. § 403(a)(1).

4. The Final Act--FDA Preamble Statements

In promulgating regulations, FDA has made clear in preambles that medical foods are not FSDU. First, in the proposed rules published in 1991 for the NLEA, FDA stated that:

> Medical foods are distinguished from the broader category of foods for special dietary use and from foods that make health claims (e.g., fiber in relation to cancer) by the requirement that medical foods be used under medical supervision. In general, to be considered a medical food,

> a product must, at a minimum meet the following criteria: The product must be a food for oral or tube feeding; the product must be labeled for the dietary management of a specific medical disorder, disease, or condition for which there are distinctive nutritional requirements; and the product must be intended to be used under medical supervision.
>
> The term "medical foods" does not pertain to all foods fed to sick patients. Medical foods are foods that are specially formulated and processed (as opposed to a naturally occurring foodstuff used in its natural state) for the patient who is seriously ill or who requires the product as a major treatment modality. Typical medical foods are enteral nutrition products. . . . Medical foods may require special quality control procedures, adequate and appropriate directions for use, and substantiation of labeling claims. They are generally not available on the retail shelf.
>
> * * *
>
> Medical foods are not foods that are simply recommended by a physician or other health care professional as part of an overall diet designed to reduce the risk of disease or medical condition or as weight loss products.
>
> * * *
>
> FDA's traditional policy has been to regulate medical foods as foods for special dietary use. However, in light of the existing definition of foods for special dietary use and the definition of medical food that has been enacted by Congress (see 21 U.S.C. 355(c) and 360ee(b)(3)), FDA is reevaluating its policy. FDA intends to address the issue of medical foods at length in a future **Federal Register** document.

56 FR 60366, 60377-78 (Nov. 27, 1993).

In the final NLEA regulations, FDA confirmed that it would address medical foods in the future while acknowledging that its preliminary view of the category may require "clarification of the types of products that are considered to be medical foods." 58 FR 2066, 2151 (Jan. 6, 1993).

Most recently, in the Federal Register announcement relating to folate labeling, FDA stated that:

> *H. Medical Foods*
>
> A comment from a trade association that represents manufacturers of medical foods supported FDA's proposal to allow the addition of folic acid to medical foods.
>
> FDA recognizes that it is necessary and appropriate to provide for the use of folic acid in foods that are formulated to be consumed or administered enterally under the supervision of a physician and that are intended for the specific dietary management of disease conditions for which

> distinctive nutritional requirements, based on recognized scientific principles, are established by medical evaluation (medical foods). Therefore, FDA is providing for the use of folic acid in medical foods in § 172.345(f). In the proposal, FDA provided for medical foods as a subset of foods for special dietary use (see proposed § 172.345(g)). However, FDA has re-evaluated this approach and concludes that it is more consistent with the act to provide for medical foods as a separate class of products (see section 403(r)(5)(A) of the act and compare section 411(c)(3) of the act with section 5(b)(3) of the Orphan Drug Act.

61 FR 8750, 8804 (March 5, 1996).

Notwithstanding the promise of a separate set of regulations, none have yet been issued. However, there has been a realization within and outside the agency that the current status of medical foods is an "NLEA loophole" with little or no regulation other than the general misbranding and adulteration provisions.

II. TYPES OF MEDICAL FOODS

In 1992, after some study and evaluation, an FDA Task Force reported on medical foods. The Task Force identified four types of products that could be, potentially, viewed as medical foods: (1) sole source nutrition products which are complete nutritional products used to replace all other food intake; (2) oral rehydration solutions for use in replacing fluids and electrolytes lost following diarrhea or vomiting; (3) modular nutrient products containing specially selected components not intended to be complete nutritional sources but designed for the management of specific diseases and which have associated claims to effectiveness either direct or implied; and, (4) products intended for use in dietary management of inborn errors of metabolism.

1. Sole Source Nutritional Products

The largest market share of medical foods would be sole source nutritional products if FDA should eventually choose to include those products within the definition. These enteral products include such common products as Isocal® and Sustacal® (Bristol-Myers Squibb); Vivonex® (Norwich Eaton); Ensure® (Ross Laboratories); and, Precision® (Sandoz). There are many others. They are generally designed and used as nutrition for individuals on tube feedings. While not complicated products--hospitals traditionally manufactured them by putting the food sent up from the kitchen in an ordinary blender--concerns could be raised about whether particular products subject to repetitive and continuous use contain total nutritive needs and do not provide excess amounts of certain electrolytes.

In 1992, FDA estimated that these products constituted 80% of the market for medical foods should they be considered as such. The market size was estimated to be in the range of $400 million annually in 1988.

2. Oral Rehydration Formulas

This subgroup also contains a number of well-known products such as Pedialyte® (Ross Laboratories). In this country, they are generally used in infants or the elderly. FDA concerns are largely limited to issues relating to assurances that the product has an appropriate electrolyte content.

3. Disease Specific Formulas

Products could include Travasorb® Hepatic or Renal (Clintec Nutrition); Lactostrict® (Fresenius) for lactose intolerance; Amin-Aid®, Immun-Aid®, Hepatic-Aid®, and Trauma-Aid® (Kendall-McGaw Laboratories); and NephrAmine® (R& D Laboratories).

While this subgroup remains small, there is a great deal of innovation. Newer products designed to maximize the immune system can be found in stores that cater to the AIDS community (*e.g.*, IMPACT® (Sandoz)).

4. Inborn Errors of Metabolism

This last category itself has an illustrious regulatory history. Before 1972, the agency regulated phenylalanine free products designed for children with phenylketonuria, such as Lofenalac®, as drugs. In 1972, the agency announced its intention to regulate this product and any similar product as a FSDU. 37 FR 18229. In 1985, however, when the agency developed its initial infant formula regulations, Lofenalac® and all formulas represented for use by an infant with an inborn error or metabolism were regulated as exempt infant formulas. 50 FR 48183 (*see* 21 C.F.R. § 107.50).

More recently, Lorenzo's Oil® (Scientific Hospital Supplies, Ltd.) might be considered within this subgroup or as a disease specific product.

III. SCOPE OF REGULATIONS

FDA's principal concerns for medical foods relate to assurances that: (1) that labeled claims for effectiveness are substantiated by clinical data; (2) good manufacturing practices ("GMPs") are adequate to maintain and deliver the components of the product necessary to achieve the intended effect; and, (3) labeling is accurate, informative, and non-misleading for its intended audience.

1. Substantiation of Claims

For many of the subgroup of products, claims are supported by broad clinical experience and products are highly standardized. To that end, products providing nutritional support are similar to blenderized meals. Oral hydration products generally comply with standards derived from clinical experience. For these products, claim substantiation on a product specific basis makes little sense.

On the other hand, many products in the other areas, including claims to effectiveness in weaning patients' from ventilators or reducing episodes of sepsis are not only amenable to clinical substantiation but would be considered misleading by FDA without it.

2. GMPs

Adherence to GMPs is especially important for life-sustaining products that must comply with standardized formulas, such as oral rehydration products. GMPs may not even be necessary for products in the arena of sole nutritional support depending on whether there is variety in the patient's diet and how long the patient is to be maintained on the product.

3. Accurate Labeling

Even though many medical foods may be designed for prescription use only, the intervention of a learned professional does not lesson FDA's historic concern with accurate labeling. Furthermore, currently, medical foods are exempt from NLEA regulatory provisions such as nutrient content information. On the other hand, medical foods are subject to the general food labeling provisions including proper statements of identity, designation of ingredients, identification of the name and place of business of the manufacturer, and declaration of net quantity of package contents.

IV. THE FUTURE

Next week, FDA is likely to publish a notice in the Federal Register that will ask specific questions about medical foods, including what they are or should be and how they should be regulated. Industry should be prepared to respond.

FDA REGULATION OF "MEDICAL FOODS" -- AN INDUSTRY PERSPECTIVE

Stephen H. McNamara
Hyman, Phelps & McNamara, P.C.
700 Thirteenth Street, N.W., Suite 1200
Washington, D.C.

The following constitues a review of the U.S. Food and Drug Administration's (FDA's) authority and practice with respect to the regulation of "medical food" products -- from the perspective of an attorney who represents industry.

1. THE STATUTORY DEFINITION OF "MEDICAL FOOD"

In the early 1970s, FDA changed its previous regulatory practice and began to accept the premise that a formulation of nutrients could be represented to provide the special nutritional needs of a person with a disease or a medical condition without triggering drug status for the product, and, that such a product could be regulated as a food instead of a drug. One of the first regulations that accepted this view (although without any discussion of the "medical food" concept) was the food additive regulation governing the use of amino acids, now codified at 21 C.F.R. § 172.320. Paragraph (f) of this regulation authorizes the addition of amino acids to "special dietary foods that are intended for use solely under medical supervision to meet nutritional requirements in specific medical conditions." 21 C.F.R. § 172.320(f). (Emphasis added.) This text appeared as a final regulation on July 26, 1973 (38 Fed. Reg. 20036, 20039; codified at that time at 21 C.F.R. § 121.101(f)).

The quoted concept ("special dietary foods that are intended for use solely under medical supervision to meet nutritional requirements in specific medical conditions") thereafter was also used in other contexts by FDA, but it was not until 1988 that an act of Congress recognized the legal category of "medical food." This occurred in the Orphan Drug Amendments of 1988 to the Federal Food, Drug, and Cosmetic Act (FDC Act). This legislation included certain provisions concerning "medical foods," and accordingly, it also provided a definition for this class of products. This is now the most authoritative governing definition of a "medical food":

> The term "medical food" means a food which is formulated to be consumed or administered enterally under the supervision of a physician and which is intended for the specific dietary management of a disease or condition for which distinctive nutritional requirements, based on recognized scientific principles, are established by medical evaluation.

21 U.S.C. § 360ee(b)(3).

2. ADVANTAGES OF "MEDICAL FOOD" STATUS

"Medical food" status has substantial advantages with respect to the use of health-related claims in labeling. In particular:

A. Exemption from Requirements for "Health Claims"

Under regulations issued by FDA in 1993, pursuant to the Nutrition Labeling and Education Act (NLEA) of 1990, it generally is not permissible to make a "health claim" on the label or in other labeling (including brochures or leaflets) for most foods unless the claim first has been approved by a final FDA regulation. 21 C.F.R. § 101.14.

"Medical foods," however, are <u>exempt</u> from this requirement. 21 C.F.R. § 101.14(f)(2). Accordingly, a "medical food" may include "health claim" information on labels and in other labeling <u>without</u> the need to obtain FDA approval.

Of course, such labeling is not immune from FDA regulation. For example, any claim that would be "false or misleading in any particular" would cause a "medical food" product to be deemed to be "misbranded" and subject to regulatory action. 21 U.S.C. § 343(a)(1). Furthermore, a "health claim" must be distinguished from a "drug claim." "Medical foods" are not entitled to make claims that would create drug status. (In general, a claim to "cure, mitigate, treat, or prevent" any "disease" would be regarded by FDA as a drug claim. 21 U.S.C. § 321(g)(1)(B). In contrast, a claim to address a patient's special dietary needs that exist because of a disease should not be regarded as a drug claim but instead should be accepted by FDA as the type of claim that can be appropriate for a "medical food.")

B. Exemption from Requirements for "Nutrient Content Claims"

Under other regulations issued by FDA in 1993 pursuant to the NLEA, it generally is not permissible to include a "nutrient content claim" on the label or in other labeling for most foods unless the claim first has been approved by a final FDA regulation. 21 C.F.R. § 101.13. For example, FDA has asserted that under these regulations it generally is not permissible for labeling to state that a food is a "good source of omega-3 fatty acids" because no FDA nutrient content claim regulation permits such labeling statements about omega-3 fatty acids.[1]

"Medical foods," however, are exempt from the requirement that nutrient content claims must be approved by FDA before use on labels or in other labeling. 21 C.F.R. § 101.13(q)(4)(ii). Of course, any claim of this type must be truthful and not misleading, and may not constitute a drug claim.

C. Exemption From "Nutrition Labeling" Requirements

Also in 1993 pursuant to the NLEA, FDA published regulations that establish a new, mandatory standard format for "nutrition labeling" for most food products. 21 C.F.R. § 101.9. A mandatory format also has been proposed by FDA for dietary supplements. 60 Fed. Reg. 67194-67224 (December 28, 1995).

Once again, however, "medical foods" are exempt from these requirements. 21 C.F.R. § 101.9(j)(8). "Medical foods" may employ any labeling text, in any format, that is truthful and not misleading (and that does not constitute a drug claim or otherwise violate some other requirement or prohibition of law, of course) to provide useful information about their nutritional content.

1 FDA has deferred enforcement of the nutrient content claim requirements with respect to "dietary supplement" products "until after December 31, 1996." 60 Fed. Reg. 7711 (February 9, 1995).

3. INTERPRETATIVE FDA REGULATIONS

In the course of recognizing that "medical foods" are exempt from the requirements for nutrition labeling, FDA has included in its regulations a section that details the agency's interpretation of the narrow class of food products that qualify as "medical foods." 21 C.F.R. § 101.9(j)(8). This FDA regulation provides that a food qualifies as a "medical food" "only if":

> (i) It is a specially formulated and processed product (as opposed to a naturally occurring foodstuff used in its natural state) for the partial or exclusive feeding of a patient by means of oral intake or enteral feeding by tube;
>
> (ii) It is intended for the dietary management of a patient who, because of therapeutic or chronic medical needs, has limited or impaired capacity to ingest, digest, absorb, or metabolize ordinary foodstuffs or certain nutrients, or who has other special medically determined nutrient requirements, the dietary management of which cannot be achieved by the modification of the normal diet alone;
>
> (iii) It provides nutritional support specifically modified for the management of the unique nutrient needs that result from the specific disease or condition, as determined by medical evaluation;
>
> (iv) It is intended to be used under medical supervision; and
>
> (v) It is intended only for a patient receiving active and ongoing medical supervision wherein the patient requires medical care on a recurring basis for, among other things, instructions on the use of the medical food.

4. APPLICATION TO "DIETARY SUPPLEMENT"-TYPE PRODUCTS

Since passage of the Dietary Supplement Health and Education Act of 1994 (DSHEA), one of the questions frequently raised at meetings such as this is whether a product that is similar to a dietary supplement in physical form, e.g., a tablet or capsule that provides vitamins and/or minerals, might qualify as a "medical food." FDA personnel appear to be reluctant to accept that a dietary supplement-type of product might qualify as a "medical food."

For example, I have heard an FDA representative assert that a particular dietary supplement-type of product could not qualify as a medical food on the premise that (A) a similar product could also be purchased as a non-medical-food dietary supplement, and therefore, (B) the dietary management of the particular condition referenced in labeling could "be achieved by the modification of the normal diet alone," with the result that (C) the product would not satisfy the terms of the FDA's definitional regulation. 21 C.F.R. § 101.9(j)(8)(ii). It can be disputed whether such a restrictive interpretation of the Orphan Drug Amendments' definition and the FDA regulation is necessary or reasonable. There is, however, no judicial law on the point.

I have also heard an FDA representative oppose "medical food" status for a dietary supplement-type of product on the premise that a "medical food" should provide the complete dietary needs of a patient, not just supplemental needs, and, on the premise that the "medical food" concept simply was not intended to apply to a tablet of vitamins and minerals. Again, however, it can be disputed whether such a restrictive reading of the definition in the Orphan Drug Amendments and in FDA's regulations is necessary or reasonable.

Under these circumstances, obviously, it is important to read and follow the definitional statute and the FDA regulation very closely and conscientiously. Whenever a company wants to market a "medical food" product, it will be important for the product clearly and consistently to be characterized in all of its labeling and other promotional materials as an item that is intended (only) for a use that complies with the definition in the Orphan Drug Amendments and the FDA regulation.

For example, any promotion of a product for use by the general public other than patients, or, any promotion that suggests that patients themselves may decide whether they should consume the product (instead of being advised to do so by their medical supervision) would run a risk of losing the special status of "medical food." ("Ask your doctor whether this is right for you" type ads should be feasible.)

(Since "medical food" status creates an exemption from requirements that otherwise generally apply with respect to use of health claims, nutrient content claims, and nutrition labeling, both FDA and the courts are likely to maintain a strict interpretation of the "medical food" definition. In general, under customary principles of statutory construction, exemptions from public health and safety legislation such as the NLEA are strictly construed.)

5. FDA GUIDANCE TO ITS INSPECTORS

In a "compliance program" entitled "Medical Foods -- Import and Domestic," FDA has provided extended specific instructions to its inspectors for the regulation of "medical food" products. FDA Compliance Program No. 7321.002; for fiscal years 1996-1998; completion date September 30, 1998. If one intends to market a "medical food," it can, of course, be informative and helpful to review the instructions that FDA has provided to its inspectors about such products.

One of the issues presented by the compliance program, for example, concerns the legal status of a single-nutrient product. The FDA compliance program instructs inspectors, "Do not collect single ingredient nutrient products that are promoted for the treatment of specific disease states . . . under this program" (Part III, page 3). It is not clear why FDA should confine this instruction to "single ingredient" nutrient products. One would have expected the agency to say that <u>any</u> product that is "promoted for the treatment of specific disease states" is not subject to regulation under the "medical food" program but is instead a drug. It is not clear whether the text of the compliance program is intended to suggest that a "single ingredient nutrient product" cannot qualify as a "medical food" at all. It would appear that a single-ingredient product is not necessarily foreclosed from status as a proper "medical food" under the definitional criteria in the Orphan Drug Amendments and FDA's regulation. Nevertheless, FDA's apparently-intentional obscurity in this regard may tend to discourage the development of single-ingredient "medical food" products, regardless of how they are used and promoted, which may be what FDA personnel want to accomplish. (On the other hand, the FDA document does explicitly recognize that "medical foods" include products that provide "[n]utritionally incomplete formulas" (Part 3).)

6. FDA CORRESPONDENCE

FDA has recently issued correspondence concerning certain products that were being sold on the premise that they were "medical foods" but that the agency alleged did not qualify as such. It appears that some of the criteria expressed in the recent letters may be narrower than the criteria expressed in the Orphan Drug Amendments and the FDA regulations. It can be helpful to review these recent letters with care, since they provide considerable insight about current FDA enforcement policy and practice.

(Insofar as views expressed in an FDA letter go beyond the requirements that are established either by the statutory definition of "medical food" in the Orphan Drug Amendments (i.e., an act of Congress) or in the FDA regulations (which FDA would maintain have the status of law), one may take the position that such views are simply the current opinion of the FDA official whose name appears on the letter and not necessarily correct. FDA regulations state that views expressed in an FDA letter "[do] not constitute an advisory opinion, [do] not necessarily represent the formal position of FDA, and [do] not bind or otherwise obligate or commit the agency to the views expressed." 21 C.F.R. § 10.85(k). Nevertheless, one should not fool himself or herself about this supposed limitation on the legal status of an FDA letter. Letters issued by senior FDA officials may not be "law," but they merit careful attention; FDA may bring regulatory actions consistent with views expressed in letters of this type.)

The following three letters are enclosed:

A. Letter Dated November 2, 1995 to Abbott Laboratories, Ross Products Division, Concerning Two Products, Including "Ensure" (Attachment A)

Before releasing this document to the public, FDA deleted the identifying text concerning the second product, presumably because confidential information was involved. However, the identification of "Ensure" is notable -- indeed, almost startling -- because only a couple of years previously, in the FDA compliance program that immediately preceded the compliance program described above, FDA had identified "Ensure" as an example of a "medical food" that was properly "sold at retail." This 1995 letter states that "Congress established a strict standard for determining when a food is a medical food," that "medical foods" are "for diseases or conditions for which distinctive nutritional requirements have been established by medical evaluation," and that FDA interprets the phrase "distinctive nutritional requirement" "to refer to the body's requirement for specific amounts of nutrients to maintain homeostasis and sustain life; that is, the amount of each nutrient that must be available for use in the metabolic and physiological processes necessary to sustain life." (Emphasis added.)

If FDA's letter means that in order to qualify as a "medical food," a product must provide the amounts of (all?) nutrients "necessary to sustain life" for a patient, it would appear that such an interpretation would be considerably narrower than the Orphan Drug Amendments or FDA's regulations require. Whether FDA will attempt to enforce such a restrictive interpretation for other products remains to be seen. (It is possible that FDA would not be able effectively to enforce this narrow interpretation without issuing new regulations that would be subject to administrative procedures and judicial review.)

B. Second FDA Letter, Also Dated November 2, 1995, to the Perrigo Company, Similarly Rejecting "Medical Food" Status for Certain Products (Attachment B)

Among other things with respect to this letter, note that even though the products' labels contained the statement, "Use under the supervision of a physician," FDA takes the position that, "This statement alone does not make a food a medical food." FDA states, "Medical foods are not foods that are simply recommended by a physician as part of an overall diet designed to reduce the risk of a disease or medical condition or to address a particular nutritional need. They are enteral products designed to address the distinctive nutritional requirements of a particular disease or condition."

In addition, FDA states that although the products addressed by this letter were labeled for use under the supervision of a physician, "the lack of prominence of this statement on the labels . . . suggests that the supervision of a physician is not crucial to the correct use of the products." (Emphasis added.)

C. Third FDA Letter, Dated January 4, 1996, to the Perrigo Company (Attachment C)

This letter reiterates FDA's views that certain products that were labeled on the premise that they were "medical foods" did not qualify for that status, for reasons similar to the reasoning in the two previously-described letters.

7. IMPENDING FDA RULEMAKING

For several years FDA personnel have been stating that the agency intends to engage in rulemaking to provide a clearer definition of "medical food" and to impose additional requirements to assure the appropriateness and safety of medical food products that are marketed. In the "unified agenda" published in the Federal

Register of May 13, 1996 (61 Fed. Reg. 22956), FDA stated that it "is considering development of regulations for medical foods . . . to assure, among other things, the safety and effectiveness of these products, proper labeling of the nutrient content and purported uses, including adequate and appropriate directions for use, and quality control and good manufacturing practices." The agency also stated that it intended to publish an "advance notice of proposed rulemaking" in October 1996.

At the present moment (this paper is being written during the first week of November 1996), the public record of the Office of Management and Budget (OMB) reveals that the proposed text for the FDA advance notice of proposed rulemaking on "medical foods" has been forwarded to OMB for review. If OMB comments are favorable, or at least do not cause the document to be sidetracked, it would appear that an advance notice of proposed rulemaking may be published in the Federal Register in the near future. (Statements by FDA to the effect that proposed rulemaking on "medical foods" was imminent were made in the past by FDA without a document subsequently being published. Nevertheless, it does appear now that publication of an advance notice of proposed rulemaking may indeed be near.)

It should be noted that an advance notice of proposed rulemaking usually does not establish any immediate changes in law or regulatory requirements, but instead triggers a public review of issues concerning whether new requirements or other changes in existing law are in fact needed, and if so, of what type. Typically, an advance notice of proposed rulemaking does not lead directly to the issuance of new final regulations, but instead, to the subsequent publication in the Federal Register of a notice of proposed rulemaking, which would be subject to another round of public comment before a final regulation would be issued. Accordingly, although it will of course be very important to review with care any advance notice of proposed rulemaking published by FDA in the near future, and for any company that has a serious interest in these matters to file appropriate comments with FDA in response to the advance notice, such a publication may not immediately change the current provisions of law concerning medical foods, as discussed in sections 1.-6. above.

8. CONCLUSION

The concept of "medical food" is now recognized and defined by an act of Congress and by FDA regulations. Furthermore, it is clear that products that qualify as "medical foods" are exempt from requirements that otherwise would apply for FDA preclearance of health claims and nutrient content claims in labeling, and that such products also are not required to use the standard FDA nutrition labeling format.

ATTACHMENT A

Mr. Michael H. Haney
Director, Regulatory Affairs
Abbott Laboratories
Ross Products Division
625 Cleveland Avenue
Columbus, Ohio 43215-1724

Dear Mr. Haney:

This is in response to your letter dated May 19, 1995, concerning implementation of label changes for the products and "Ensure."

In your letter, you addressed two issues raised by the Food and Drug Administration (FDA) in our letter to Ross Products Division (Ross) dated April 11, 1995. First, you asserted that the institutional line of Ensure products are intended for use as a medical food, and thus, are exempt from nutrition labeling and that you intend to defer taking steps to re-label these products until after a meeting with FDA.

While we are willing to meet with representatives of Ross and Abbott Laboratories, we believe that it is important that we first clearly articulate the agency's interpretation of the requirements of the Federal Food, Drug, and Cosmetic Act (the act) with regard to the regulation of foods for special dietary use and medical foods. After you have considered these views, you can decide whether you still wish to meet with us.

We retain a basic disagreement with you as to whether Ensure is a medical food. Underlying our disagreement is a fundamental difference in view as to what a medical food is. Your letter reflects the view that to be a medical food, it is enough that a manufacturer label the product to be a medical food and intend that the product meet the distinctive nutritional requirements of a disease or condition, regardless of whether there is any evidence that such distinctive nutritional requirements exist or that the product, as formulated and consumed, actually meets those requirements, assuming that they do exist.

We believe that the act establishes the need for substantiation for a medical food's claimed usefulness in the dietary management of disease. The statute establishes a range of circumstances in which claims relating to a disease may be made. At one end of the spectrum is a conventional food, which under section 403(r) may bear a health claim if the scientific validity of the health claim is supported by significant scientific agreement. At the other end of the spectrum is a drug, whose effectiveness in curing, treating, mitigating, or preventing disease must be established by substantial evidence. Clearly, a medical food falls within this spectrum. In defining a medical food in the Orphan Drug Act, Congress included the requirement that distinctive nutritional requirements of a disease or condition exist, and that they be established by medical evaluation and meet accepted scientific standards. Thus, Congress established a strict standard for determining when a food is a medical food. It is inconceivable that the statute should not also be interpreted as establishing a similarly strict standard for determining whether the medical food meets the distinctive nutritional requirements of the patient for whom it was formulated.

However, your position that the manufacturer intend the product to meet the special needs of the disease would establish a subjective standard that requires little more than the manufacturer's statement of intent. The inappropriateness of your view is underscored by the distinction between a food for special dietary use and a medical food, which you do not address in your letter.

Medical foods are for diseases or conditions for which distinctive nutritional requirements have been established by medical evaluation. While the law does not define what constitutes a "distinctive nutritional requirement," we interpret this phrase to refer to the body's requirement for specific amounts of nutrients to maintain homeostasis and sustain life; that is, the amount of each nutrient that must be available for use in the metabolic and physiological processes necessary to sustain life.

The nutritional requirements of healthy people for specific nutrients reflect the quantitative and qualitative requirements for absorbed nutrients (i.e., the physiologic requirement) with adjustments for common inefficiencies associated with absorption, utilization, and retention. However, the dietary management of patients with specific diseases requires, in some instances, the ability to meet nutritional requirements that differ substantially from the needs of healthy persons. For example, in establishing the Recommended Dietary Allowances for the general, healthy population, the Food and Nutrition Board recognized, that different or distinctive physiologic requirements may need to be met for certain persons with "special nutritional needs arising from metabolic disorders, chronic diseases, injuries, premature birth, other medical conditions, and drug therapies,[1]" compared to the amount of nutrient needed in otherwise healthy persons to support life or maintain homeostasis. Thus, the distinctive nutritional needs associated with a disease would reflect the total requirement needed by a healthy person, adjusted for the distinctive changes in the nutritional needs of the patient due to the effect of the disease process on metabolism, absorption, or excretion. These distinctive nutritional requirements, which may be greater than, less than, or in a narrower range of tolerance than for an otherwise healthy individual, are the distinctive nutritional requirements that define a medical food.

Medical foods, therefore, are formulated to aid in the dietary management of a disease or health-related condition that presents distinctive nutritional requirements that are different from the nutritional requirements of otherwise healthy people. In contrast to medical foods,

---

[1]Food and Nutrition Board, Recommended Dietary Allowances, 10th ed., National Academy Press, Washington, D.C., 1989.

there are foods that are specially formulated to provide only the dietary requirements consistent with recommendations for the general population. These foods are foods for special dietary use. Dietary requirements do not reflect a nutritional problem per se; that is, the physiological requirements for nutrients necessary to maintain life or homeostasis addressed by such foods are similar to those of normal, healthy persons. These foods are formulated in such a way that only the ingredients or physical form of the diet is different. The quantitative and qualitative nutrient requirements of the person consuming these foods are not significantly different from those of the general population. For example, a person who has difficulty swallowing solid food may have a special dietary need for a food that is in liquid form, but this special dietary need doesn't change his physiologic nutrient requirements. Similarly, a person with a gluten-sensitive enteropathy requires specially formulated protein in the diet that doesn't contain gluten; however, the actual amounts of protein (i.e., amino acids) required by the body is not different than in otherwise healthy persons. Thus, foods for special dietary use are intended to meet ordinary nutritional requirements through special dietary means.

Therefore, for a product to be a medical food, rather than a food for special dietary use, it must be intended for a disease for which there are distinctive nutritional requirements, and the product must be shown to meet those requirements. We note that the requirement that the disease be one that creates distinctive nutritional requirements creates a very high standard, one that is met by only a relatively few diseases (hence the inclusion of the definition of "medical food" as part of the Orphan Drug Act). You have not shown that Ensure is intended to meet the distinctive nutritional requirements of such a disease. Thus, Ross has not met the fundamental requirement for qualifying a product as a medical food.

The agency is willing to meet with representatives of Ross concerning the issues raised in this letter and our letters of March 2, March 22, and April 11, 1995. If you wish to meet with us in regard to the labeling of Ensure, you should contact us as soon as possible to arrange a meeting.

The agency has carefully reviewed the revised labels for Ensure and that you submitted with your letter and offer the following comments concerning them.

Ensure.

> The nutrition label of Ensure does not meet the leading and type size requirements of § 101.9(d)(1)(ii)(C) and (d)(1)(iii), respectively, and the hairlines required by § 101.9(d)(1)(v) are missing under the listing of calories and dietary fiber and between the lines of vitamins and minerals. As noted above, if it is technologically infeasible or impracticable to meet these requirements, Ross may write to the Office of Food Labeling and request permission to deviate from the regulations under § 101.9(g)(9). When making such a request, the firm should clearly identify all products for which the request is being made; include a sample container, when appropriate; state why it is technologically infeasible or impracticable to adhere to the regulations; and identify the alternative means of compliance that would be used to provide the nutrition information (e.g., specify the size of type and leading to be used).

We hope this information adequately addresses the issues you raised. If we can be of further assistance, please contact us.

Sincerely yours,

Elizabeth A. Yetley, Ph.D., R.D.
Director
Office of Special Nutritionals
Center for Food Safety
and Applied Nutrition

ATTACHMENT B

Mr. Mike Jandernoa
Chairman and CEO
Perrigo Company
117 Water Street
Allegan, Michigan 49010

Dear Mr. Jandernoa:

This letter is to inform you that the Food and Drug Administration (FDA) has reviewed the labels for the products "Good Sense Nutritional Supplement Plus," "DailySource Nutritional Supplement," and "DailySource Nutritional Supplement Plus" and has determined that the labels for these products do not meet the nutrition labeling requirements of section 403 of the Federal Food, Drug, and Cosmetic Act (the Act). The specific problems noted by FDA are described below.

FDA has reviewed the labels for the products identified above and has determined that these products are not medical foods as defined in section 5(b) of the Orphan Drug Act (21 U.S.C. 360ee(b)(3)) and do not qualify for the exemption in 21 USC 343(q)(5)(A) from the nutrition labeling requirements in 21 USC 343(q) and 21 CFR 101.9. Good Sense Nutritional Supplement Plus, DailySource Nutritional Supplement, and DailySource Nutritional Supplement Plus are, therefore, misbranded under 21 USC 343(q).

The labels of Good Sense Nutritional Supplement Plus, DailySource Nutritional Supplement, and DailySource Nutritional Supplement Plus state that these products can be used "To help stay healthy, energetic, active;" as a "Meal replacement or supplement;" and to "Gain or maintain healthy weight." The statement "To help stay healthy, energetic, active" evidences that the product is intended for use by healthy people, and that it is not a "food which is formulated to be consumed or administered enterally under the supervision of a physician and which is intended for the specific dietary management of a disease or condition for which distinctive nutritional requirements, based on recognized scientific principles, are established by medical evaluation;" that is, that it is not a medical food (see

21 USC 360ee(b)(3)). Medical foods are foods intended for the dietary management of a patient receiving active and ongoing medical supervision. At a minimum, under the statutory definition, to be considered a medical food, a product must be for enteral use; must be labeled for the dietary management of a specific medical disorder, disease, or condition for which there are distinctive nutritional requirements; and must be intended for use under medical supervision (see 21 CFR 101.9(j)(8)(ii), (iii), and (v)). The labels of Good Sense Nutritional Supplement Plus, DailySource Nutritional Supplement, and DailySource Nutritional Supplement Plus do not evidence that the products are intended for the dietary management of any specific medical disorder, disease, or condition. This fact, and the fact that the labels use the words "stay healthy," demonstrate that the products are intended for use by persons without a medical disorder, disease, or condition for which distinctive nutritional requirements exist. Therefore, Good Sense Nutritional Supplement Plus, DailySource Nutritional Supplement, and DailySource Nutritional Supplement Plus are not medical foods.

Although your labels contain the statement "Use under the supervision of a physician," this statement alone does not make a food a medical food. Medical foods are not foods that are simply recommended by a physician as part of an overall diet designed to reduce the risk of a disease or medical condition or to address a particular nutritional need. They are enteral products designed to address the distinctive nutritional requirements of a particular disease or condition.

Moreover, the statement that a product is intended for use under the supervision of a physician is intended to inform patients that the product is for the dietary management of a patient who is receiving active and ongoing medical supervision, and that the patient should only use the product while continuing to receive care and instruction from a physician. This statement should be prominent so as to convey this message to the consumer and to encourage compliance. The lack of prominence of this statement on the labels of Good Sense Nutritional Supplement Plus, DailySource Nutritional Supplement, and DailySource Nutritional Supplement Plus, particularly when compared to the prominence given the instructions for the use of the products, suggests that the supervision of a physician is not crucial to the correct use of the products.

The labels also state that Good Sense Nutritional Supplement Plus, DailySource Nutritional Supplement, and DailySource Nutritional Supplement Plus are for "Meal replacement or supplement" and to "Gain or maintain healthy weight." As the definition of "medical food" makes clear, medical foods are not foods that are simply recommended by a physician as part of an overall diet designed to help weight loss or maintenance.

Based on the statements in their labeling, Good Sense Nutritional Supplement Plus, DailySource Nutritional Supplement, and DailySource Nutritional Supplement Plus are foods for special dietary use. As such, these products are subject to the labeling requirements in 21 CFR Parts 101 and 105. Because Good Sense Nutritional Supplement Plus, DailySource Nutritional Supplement, and DailySource Nutritional Supplement Plus fail to comply with 21 CFR Part 101 and the underlying provisions of the Act in several significant respects, they are misbranded food.

The labels of the products Good Sense Nutritional Supplement Plus, DailySource Nutritional Supplement, and DailySource Nutritional Supplement Plus are in violation of section 403 of the act as follows:

> The labels fail to bear nutrition labeling in accordance with 21 CFR 101.9.
>
> The labels contain various nutrient content claims such as "250 Calories," "355 Calories," and "fortified" that are not made in a manner that is consistent with the definitions or requirements in 21 CFR 101.13 and Part 101 Subpart D for use of these terms.

The above identification of violations is not intended to be an all-inclusive list of deficiencies in the labeling of your products. It is your responsibility to assure adherence with all requirements of the Act.

The Perrigo Company should take prompt action to correct these deficiencies in the labeling of Good Sense Nutritional Supplement Plus, DailySource Nutritional Supplement, and DailySource Nutritional Supplement Plus. Within 15 working days identify the changes the Perrigo Company intends to make in the labels of Good Sense Nutritional Supplement Plus, DailySource Nutritional Supplement, and DailySource Nutritional Supplement Plus. We also ask that the Perrigo Company provide the agency with copies of the new labels for these products. Continued marketing of these products bearing labels that do not meet applicable mandatory nutrition labeling requirements may result in regulatory action.

Your reply should be sent to the Food and Drug Administration, Office of Special Nutritionals, HFS-450, 200 C Street, S.W., Washington, DC 20204. If there are any questions, they may be directed to Nicholas Duy who is available by phone at (202) 205-5372.

Sincerely yours,

Elizabeth A. Yetley, Ph.D., R.D.
Acting Director
Office of Special Nutritionals
Center for Food Safety
and Applied Nutrition

ATTACHMENT C

Ms. Heidi Horn
Regulatory Affairs Manager
Perrigo Company
117 Water Street
Allegan, Michigan 49010

Dear Ms. Horn:

This is in response to your letter dated November 29, 1995, responding to concerns raised by the Food and Drug Administration (FDA) in our letter to Perrigo Company, dated November 2, 1995, about the labeling of the products "Good Sense Nutritional Supplement Plus," "DailySource Nutritional Supplement," and "DailySource Nutritional Supplement Plus."

We have carefully considered the information contained in your letter and recognize the substantial effort that Perrigo has made to correct the label deficiencies that we described in our November 2, 1995 letter. However, in your letter, you raised two issues that we believe should be addressed in more detail by the agency than they were in our previous letter. First, although you indicated that you would take steps to relabel your products in accordance with the provisions of 21 CFR 101.9, you appear to disagree with our explanation about the types of products eligible for an exemption from nutrition labeling under the provisions of 21 CFR 101.9(j)(8). Second, you also indicated that you did not agree with FDA's statement that the declaration of the calorie content on the label (e.g., outside of the nutrition facts box) is a nutrient content claim. We address each of this issues below.

The agency believes that in order for a food to be deemed to be a medical food, it must meet the statutory definition of a medical food as set forth in the section 5(b) of the Orphan Drug Act (21 U.S.C. 360ee(b)). In our view, there is a fundamental difference between medical food and foods for special dietary use.

Medical foods are for diseases or conditions for which distinctive nutritional requirements have been established by medical evaluation. While the law does not define what constitutes a "distinctive nutritional requirement," we interpret this phrase to refer to the body's requirement for specific amounts of nutrients to maintain homeostasis and sustain life; that is, the amount of each nutrient that must be available for use in the metabolic and physiological processes necessary to sustain life.

The nutritional requirements of healthy people for specific nutrients reflect the quantitative and qualitative requirements for absorbed nutrients (i.e., the physiologic requirement) with adjustments for common inefficiencies associated with absorption, utilization, and retention. However, the dietary management of patients with specific diseases requires, in some instances, the ability to meet nutritional requirements that differ substantially from the needs of healthy persons. For example, in establishing the Recommended Dietary Allowances for the general, healthy population, the Food and Nutrition Board recognized, that different or distinctive physiologic requirements may need to be met for certain persons with "special nutritional needs arising from metabolic disorders, chronic diseases, injuries, premature birth, other medical conditions, and drug therapies,[1]" compared to the amount of nutrient needed in otherwise healthy persons to support life or maintain homeostasis. Thus, the distinctive nutritional needs associated with a disease would reflect the total requirement needed by a healthy person, adjusted for the distinctive changes in the nutritional needs of the patient due to the effect of the disease process on metabolism, absorption, or excretion. These distinctive nutritional requirements, which may be greater than, less than, or in a narrower range of tolerance than for an otherwise healthy individual, are the distinctive nutritional requirements that define a medical food.

Medical foods, therefore, are formulated to aid in the dietary management of a disease or health-related condition that presents distinctive nutritional requirements that are different from the nutritional requirements of otherwise healthy people. In contrast to medical foods, there are foods that are specially formulated to provide only the dietary requirements consistent with recommendations for the general population. These foods are foods for

[1]Food and Nutrition Board, Recommended Dietary Allowances, 10th ed., National Academy Press, Washington, D.C., 1989.

special dietary use. Dietary requirements do not reflect a nutritional problem *per se*; that is, the physiological requirements for nutrients necessary to maintain life or homeostasis addressed by such foods are similar to those of normal, healthy persons. These foods are formulated in such a way that only the ingredients or physical form of the diet is different. The quantitative and qualitative nutrient requirements of the person consuming these foods are not significantly different from those of the general population. For example, a person who has difficulty swallowing solid food may have a special dietary need for a food that is in liquid form, but this special dietary need doesn't change his physiologic nutrient requirements. Similarly, a person with a gluten-sensitive enteropathy requires specially formulated protein in the diet that doesn't contain gluten; however, the actual amount of protein (i.e., amino acids) required by the body is not different than in otherwise healthy persons. Thus, foods for special dietary use are intended to meet ordinary nutritional requirements through special dietary means.

Therefore, for a product to be a medical food, rather than a food for special dietary use, it must be intended for a disease for which there are distinctive nutritional requirements, and the product must be shown to meet those requirements. We note that the requirement that the disease be one that creates distinctive nutritional requirements creates a very high standard, one that is met by only a relatively few diseases (hence the inclusion of the definition of "medical food" as part of the Orphan Drug Act). Since Perrigo has not shown that their products are intended to meet the distinctive nutritional requirements of such a disease, you have not met the fundamental requirement for qualifying a product as a medical food.

The second issue that you raise concerns whether a statement or declaration of the calorie content of a food on the label constitutes a nutrient content claim. You maintain that a statement such as "250 calories" made on a label outside of the Nutrition Facts box is not a nutrient content claim. We disagree. The agency considers all statements authorized by 21 CFR 101.13(i) which "contain a statement about the amount or percentage of a nutrient," including statements such as this, to be nutrient content claims.

Specifically, 21 CFR 101.13(c) states that information required or permitted by 21 CFR 101.9 to be declared in nutrition labeling, and that appears as part of the nutrition labeling, is not a nutrient content claim. However, if such information is declared elsewhere on the label or in labeling, it is a nutrient content claim and is subject to the requirements for nutrient content claims, including the requirements for referral statements.

If you have questions about either of the issues discussed above, please contact Dr. Robert Moore, Office of Special Nutritionals, HFS-456, 200 C Street, S.W., Washington, D.C. 20204 (telephone (202) 205-4605 or 5372).

Sincerely yours,

Elizabeth A. Yetley, Ph.D., R.D.
Director
Office of Special Nutritionals
Center for Food Safety
and Applied Nutrition

WHAT IS SUFFICIENT EVIDENCE TO SUPPORT A HEALTH-MEDICAL CLAIM?

Stephen L. DeFelice, M.D.
The Foundation For Innovation in Medicine
Cranford
New Jersey

The primary objective of FIM is to create a system which dramatically encourages nutraceutical research. The problem has been, and to a much lesser extent remains, the absence of a system that justifies the investment required to make nutraceutical claims. The good news is that, despite present barriers, the regulatory category "medical foods", "foods," under the Nutrition Labeling & Education Act (NLEA) and "dietary supplements" as defined by the Dietary Supplement Health & Education Act (DSHEA) have had a major impact both on the market environment and the will of corporations to conduct nutraceutical research. Briefly put, **the present U.S. system now makes it economically feasible for companies to conduct preclinical and clinical research and to make health-medical claims.**

The great societal question is "What is sufficient evidence to make a nutraceutical health-medical claim?" (FIM maintains that there is little or no difference between a health claim or medical claim. Attempts to separate the two are confusing having a negative impact on nutraceutical research.) The answer is there is no magic formula or standard. For this reason, historically, government created standards that allowed it, and not the physician-scientist community, to decide what is sufficient evidence for efficacy and safety claims for drugs, devices, biologics, etc. NLEA states that **there must be significant scientific agreement** to justify FDA's approval of a health-medical claim for a food. But significant scientific agreement simply does not exist as a definable entity. Whether it exists at all once more depends on an arbitrary decision made by the government, the FDA.

And now the new dilemma: Under DSHEA (dietary supplements) and the medical foods categories, it is the company and not a government body that decides what is sufficient evidence to make a health-medical claim. This presents an enormous challenge, for there are no established standards or guidelines which define what is sufficient evidence to justify such claims.

It is imperative to expeditiously establish and implement guidelines to characterize the nature of such evidence in order to ensure that the resulting benefit to society will far outweigh the risk. FIM believes that the issue which best addresses the societal benefit-to-risk ratio is based on the need to dramatically increase nutraceutical research, particularly, clinical nutraceutical research.

FIM'S GUIDELINES FOR SUFFICIENT EVIDENCE FOR NUTRACEUTICAL (HEALTH-MEDICAL) CLAIMS

1. **There must be sufficient clinical data to support the claim.** (The studies need not be double-blind.)

2. **Acceptable surrogate markers (instead of clinical endpoints) can be sufficient to support a claim.**

3. **Acceptable preclinical data to support the product rationale are desirable but not always necessary.**

4. **All pertinent data must be published in respected medical-scientific journals.** (This is the first step of the peer review process.)

5. **Independent consensus or expert group opinion should be obtained.** (This is the second step of the peer review process.)

6. **Post-marketing surveillance.** This effort should concentrate particularly on the aspect of safety.

As with all things in life, FIM's guidelines are imperfect. One can argue that clever charlatans can successfully weave their way through such guidelines. But this is true in all systems of life. Even with the high standards of research studies (including the "gold standard", controlled, randomized double-blind clinical trials) conducted by ethical companies and required by FDA for NDA approved drugs are not foolproof. For example, finasteride was approved by the FDA for the indication of benign prostatic hypertrophy. A recent study, however, reported that the clinical benefit of this product may be much more limited than that of the original FDA approved indication. Extensively researched, NDA- approved short-acting calcium-channel blockers drugs have recently been reported to increase the incidence of cardiovascular deaths and perhaps increase the incidence of cancer. Even the lipid-lowering drugs, the statins, where the data to reduce cardiovascular events are promising, have not passed the full test of proof. These products are recommended to be taken for a lifetime. The current data are far from lifetime data, and one would not be surprised if some significant adverse effects occurred after more prolonged and extensive use of these drugs. The conclusion is that even with volumes of peer reviewed data in journals, rigorously examined by the FDA and its consultants, one can never be sure regarding the total efficacy and safety of drug products in common use.

With nutraceutical data, we also have the same problems. Based on the data in approximately one dozen publications, it was not unreasonable to assume that beta-carotene might be effective in the prevention of lung cancer. In fact, many qualified health professionals recommended supplementation with beta-carotene in high-risk patients. Then a controlled, prospective double-blind clinical trial reported no beneficial clinical effect (and possibly a negative one) on lung cancer. What is the truth? Many experts still believe that the answer is not yet known.

Even under NLEA, which grants the FDA authority to decide what determines significant scientific agreement to support a claim for a food, most of the claims approved by the agency are based on data that fall far short of those typically required for a drug. Nor is the "five vegetable-fruit portions per day diet" recommended by the National Cancer Institute (NCI) to prevent cancer supported by well-controlled, double-blind clinical trials. Though there is wisdom in such claims and recommendations, they are not substantiated by controlled clinical trials.

In conclusion, our society, including the FDA, has already begun to accept the reality that the amount of evidence to support a health-medical claim should and does not necessarily require double-blind, controlled clinical trials.

A SPECIAL NOTE ON SAFETY

One would not be surprised if, in the future, a major nutraceutical tragedy were to occur. What is surprising, however, is that it has not yet occurred. Millions of Americans consume large amounts of all types of potential remedies with little data to support the clinical benefits and safety of the vast majority of them. It is indeed puzzling why we have not seen more obvious examples of toxic or adverse effects.

FIM's nutraceutical guidelines address data on both efficacy and safety and will help to identify and perhaps decrease harmful effects. Companies, under present law, will have the right to educate consumers, physicians and other health professionals about such data. **FIM firmly believes that good products supported by good data that are available to all, will drive out bad products.**

There is emerging a class of dietary supplement products that are perceived to carry particularly high risks. Melatonin and DHEA are two such examples. FIM believes it is particularly important to devise ways to handle such potentially high risk products, as long as they do not discourage nutraceutical research. For example, a system that attempts to excessively control such products might have prevented the research and availability of folic acid, vitamin E, calcium and fiber and might also prevent the advent of valuable nutraceuticals.

For the survival of a vigorous research-driven nutraceutical system, something must be done to adequately control potentially high-risk products in commerce. One major catastrophe can lead to legislation that would dramatically decrease research incentives. Though difficult to do well, some type of tracking system should be established to assess such risk and, if found, to limit it. It could be done by some government body.

MEDICAL FOODS: WHAT IS SUFFICIENT EVIDENCE TO SUPPORT A HEALTH-MEDICAL CLAIM?

Louis Lasagna, M.D.
Sackler School of Graduate Biomedical Sciences
Tufts University
Boston, MA

The following represents a nutraceutical analogue of the 95 theses posted on the door of the Wittenberg Castle church on October 31, 1517 in the start of the Reformation. There are, I am happy to report, only 12, and they represent the basic postulates of an aging clinical pharmacologist whose experience is greater with respect to drugs than foods, but who believes it not a coincidence that from earliest times, foods and drugs have been regulated together in different countries.

I. Certain nutraceutical substances have clearly demonstrated their ability to prevent or ameliorate some pathological processes. Folic acid to prevent spina bifida and cranberry juice to prevent urinary tract infections are two examples, but many others could be given.

II. On the other hand, certain substances are being consumed by the public whose medical ability is not as yet clearly proven. Melatonin, e.g., has hypnotic properties but its ability to prevent aging, cancers, etc., as some believe, has been promoted (as in the popular book "The Melatonin Miracle") in a way that reminds one of the past excesses and hyperbole of the snake oil salesman of the last century.

III. Both the lay public and the medical profession have, within their ranks, significant numbers of people who are interested in (and taking) nutraceuticals to prevent or treat disease.

IV. It is needlessly confusing and intellectually futile to seek distinctions between "health claims" and "medical claims." To do so serves only to gladden the heart of Lewis Carroll's ghost. We do not need to walk "Through the Looking Glass" into Wonderland.

V. "Significant scientific agreement" defies operational definition. When FDA approves a medicine after a 7 - 6 vote by an agency advisory committee, is that "significant scientific agreement" or "significant scientific disagreement"? In point of fact, disagreement among experts is not at all rare, which is why Senator Eastland's subcommittee, as part of the legislative history of the 1962 Kefauver-Harris Amendments, asserted that a drug deemed safe and effective by a minority of qualified professionals should be approved for marketing.

VI. A decision made by the FDA to approve a drug (and I would think of a nutraceutical as well) always represents a judgment call -- to wit, that if used as labeled, the substance will do a lot more good than harm. "Safe and effective" never means safe for all individuals or effective for all individuals.

VII. If corporate sponsors are to be allowed to decide when evidence exists of sufficient quality and quantity to make a medical claim, they must invoke the aid of independent experts to evaluate the data and render an opinion as to their merits. These experts must not be robotically narrow. They should be willing to consider any and all available evidence -- animal data, "naturalistic" experience, epidemiologic data, randomized controlled trials, case control studies, surrogate markers, etc. As Sir Austin Bradford Hill, one of the original leaders in controlled trial methodology pointed out 30 years ago, "any belief that the controlled trial is the only way [to study therapeutic efficacy] would mean not that the pendulum had swung too far, but that it had come right off its hook." (Remember that some of our most important public health tenets, such as cholesterol and coronary heart disease risk, or cigarette smoking and emphysema and lung cancer, came from epidemiologic data.)

Useful data may or may not have been published, and if published may or may not have appeared in peer-reviewed journals, but clearly peer-reviewed and peer-accepted articles will usually weigh more heavily in the balance.

VIII. The implementation of all the above should be approached flexibly, taking into account the seriousness and importance of the specific health issue, the existence of alternative substitutes, and safety issues. FDA has shown its willingness to grant approval for cancer and AIDS treatment, e.g., on the basis of much less data than would ordinarily be required for approval by the agency.

IX. Rare serious adverse events may surface for the first time only after substantial experience in the population. These are usually not predictable from animal studies or the amount of clinical data ordinarily available prior to registration. Even with a cautious agency like the FDA, 3% of approved new chemical entities are eventually withdrawn from the market because of the appearance of serious, previously unexpected adverse events. There is a need, therefore, for post-marketing surveillance, but we must not be paralyzed by fears about adverse events. As Clarke has said, "The unknown is not a wrinkle to be ironed out of the social fabric."

X. History teaches us that yesterday's scorned hypothesis is tomorrow's accepted truth. (I can remember when the Shute brothers in Canada were considered foolish for espousing Vitamin E for its beneficial cardiovascular effects.)

XI. Agnosticism is not an option with regard to nutraceuticals. If, e.g., you decide to follow the NCI's vegetable-fruit dietary recommendations (as yet unsubstantiated by persuasive data), you are betting that you will benefit therefrom. If you don't follow the recommendations, you are betting that benefits will not accrue to you. There is no position that amounts to a postponement of judgment.

XII. Finally, let me argue that when a medical claim is first proposed for a nutraceutical, such claim is then and there either true or false. What subsequently gathered data provide are persuasion and quantification -- persuasion aimed either at disbelievers and skeptics, or devotees and adherents, and intended to convince people to accept the claim as true or reject it as false, and quantification aimed at describing how much benefit and harm are likely to ensue from use of the nutraceutical.

Aspirin, e.g., was not subjected to controlled modern trials until the 1980s, but salicylates had been providing pain relief and anti-inflammatory benefits for centuries. Aspirin did not "become" an analgesic because of controlled trials.

MEDICAL FOODS: THE EUROPEAN APPROACH

Gérard Pilley

Chief Executive Officer
GRAND PUBLIC S. A.
42, Avenue Montaigne
75008 PARIS
Tél. : 01 53 67 52 44 - Télécopie 01 53 67 52 45

Before getting to the heart of the matter, I would like to thank Dr. DeFelice. We have supported each other since the beginning of our crusade in favor of Nutraceuticals, a word that he created and that I then introduced for the first time in France 10 years ago when translating Steve's book.

A second comment deals with my late arrival to this conference due to a reason that certainly might be of interest to you. I was retained in Paris by a particularly fascinating Nutraceutical product or a Medical Food that won the Innovation gold medal at the « Food Ingredient Europe 1996 » symposium.

This product is an egg. A hen egg with the trademark Omegatech imprinted on its shell, Omegatech being the company in Boulder, Colorado that, in a way, invented it.

This egg contains 150 mg of DHA and, considering that the fish-oil medication that I developed in France some years ago under the brand name Maxepa® contains 120 mg of DHA by capsule, I thought I should not encounter too much difficulty in supporting a health allegation for Omegatech eggs.

But the question is: is it a Medical Food, a Functional Food, or a Nutraceutical?

This semantic problem appears here and there in Europe, and specifically in France; we are far from reaching a consensus.

Some people do not want to hear about Nutraceuticals because they associate them with essentially marketing inventions that are likely to turn out to be charlatanism. However, often they do not know the precise definition of the word Nutraceutical, at least as it is defined by the Foundation for Innovation in Medicine.

Other people do not like the term Medical Foods, which too often raises the possibility that these products will be classified in the monopoly of pharmacists (in many European countries, this monopoly is protected by law), and they fear the establishment of too strict regulation by health authorities.

I would like to offer another comment on the allegation made earlier in the conference room, that there is no nutraceutical market in Europe. I believe that it does exist, but that there is no detectable specific nutraceutical category and that no nutraceutical industry can be clearly visualized. Nevertheless, the number of products belonging to the nutraceutical class is increasing daily in many categories and through all the distribution networks: supermarkets, hypermarkets, stores that sell personal hygiene products, health shops, and even pharmacies.

These products are often developed by large food-processing companies, of which it can no longer be said that their investments in Research & Development are too weak.

The number of products is actually growing very rapidly. To illustrate, I would point out that, some days ago, Danone Group (one of the largest food-processing companies in the world) created, through its Research Institute, an annual $200,000 prize to reward an innovation in the field of Nutrition and Health.

Finally, I must recognize the relevance of the remark made by my peer from Sigmatau: that the excess of promotion—in the United States—of products that strictly speaking are not foodstuffs but that can be found in supermarkets (for example, melatonin, DHEA, and herbal ecstasy) leads to considerable adverse publicity and nourishes authorities' suspicions, thus harming honest and « reasonable » companies.

Now let me provide you with an overall view of the Medical Foods regulatory environment. I will describe this first for France and then for Europe, because Europe is still waiting for a regulation for which the constitutive elements are not forecast according to a precise deadline. Also, there are many sections in the European regulations that each member state must transpose into its own legislation, but the opposite movement can also occur. Each member state actually manages the problem of Medical Foods according to its own scheme; concerning the latter, Germany and the United Kingdom are more advanced than their neighboring countries.

Now let us consider the main enactments and regulatory texts that provide the framework for Foods and Medical Foods.

FRANCE

A. Decree of 07.12.1984

The Consumer's Code, in its decree of 07.12.1984 on truthful information on foodstuffs, is the transposition of the European directive EEC 84/450.

This text defines a foodstuff and prohibits any reference that indicates that the foodstuff possesses particular characteristics (even if all similar foodstuffs possess these same characteristics) and also prohibits claims of preventative properties, treatment and healing of human illnesses, and claims of evoking such properties.

B. Decree of 17.05.1989

A notice on 17.05.1989 from the CEDAP (Interministerial Commission On Products For a Special Diet) regulates the mixing of nutrients for special liquid foodstuffs. These products fall into two categories:

- balanced nutritious mixes
- dietary nutritious mixes

The first group has the following characteristics:

- proteins of 12–13% of their total caloric value, with a chemical index either equal to or above 80.
- lipids of 20–35% with at least 4% of triglycerides in cis-cis form.
- glucide 47–68%
- minerals and vitamins—tables are provided of their amounts in each element

The second group, dietary mixes, are unbalanced and their first definition is that they are different from those in the first group. The formulas for them are very detailed, and the justification for their recommendation for certain groups of the population must be established scientifically and then through clinical studies.

Certain substances added to these mixes are included in the positive list (regulation of 01.07.1976).

Overall, it can be said that balanced mixes are for consumption by healthy people who need such nutrition on a temporary basis, for example, after undergoing surgery. In contrast, the unbalanced mixes are for those requiring a particular kind of nutrition.

C. Notice of 01.07.1976

An important notice issued on 01.07.1976 covers foods for newborn babies (0–1 year) and for young children (1–3 years). Chapters 1 to 4 of this text cover normal feeding, while Chapter 5 addresses problems arising with children who have metabolic problems or particular nutritional requirements.

The labeling must indicate the nature of the problem and carry the warning "not to be used without medical advice."

D. Decree of 29.08.1991

Decree number 91-827 of 29.08.1991 regulates and defines foodstuffs for particular dietary needs. These are for people with absorption or metabolic problems, those who have certain physiological conditions, or infants and young children in good health.

The labeling of these products, the nine subcategories of which can be found in Appendix A, is extremely detailed.

E. TIPS

There is a special procedure, TIPS (Interministerial Tariff for Health Benefits), that allows for financial charges through the social security system for certain groups of nutrients (mixes, proteins, glucides, triglycerides, single proteins, or single lipids) currently aimed at two categories of illness:

- those suffering from mucovicidosis (cystic fibrosis)
- those infected with HIV, in whom malnutrition is characterized by loss of over 5% of body weight

EUROPE

A. EU Directive 79/112

The EU directive 79/112 of 18.12.1978 is aimed at harmonizing the legislation, labeling, presentation and advertising of food commodities.

NB: general food products must not in any way allude to particular properties or the prevention or treatment of human illnesses.

B. EU Directive 84/450

As has been seen previously in French law, the EU directive 84/450 of 10.09. 1984 harmonizes the texts in order to prevent any breach of truthful information to consumers. It also prohibits any allusion to prevention or treatment of human illnesses.

C. EU Directive 89/398

The EU directive 89/398 of 03.05.1989 proposes the harmonization of legislation for all food commodities for specific dietary requirements (a new denomination of dietary products).

These products are for certain groups of people, as has been illustrated in French law: those with absorption or metabolic problems or particular physiological needs, or young children in good health.

It will be noted that this directive foresees the possibility that a member state will contest the classification of such a product on the basis of detailed scientific evidence.

D. EU Directive 90/496

EU directive 90/496, dated 24.09.1990, regulates, both qualitatively and quantitatively, the labeling of normal food products and their nutritional content.

E. STAN 180/1991

I would now like to draw attention to part of the *Codex Alimentarius* STAN 180/1991, which is, of course, submitted to each of the member states of the European Union.

I would also like to take this opportunity to thank Dr. Dominique Baelde of the French delegation to the *Codex Alimentarius*, and to acknowledge the presence of Dr. Elizabeth Yetley, who is the U.S. representative to this body.

I would briefly remind you that the *Codex Alimentarius* is an international body formed by the World Health Organization and the Food and Agriculture Organization. The plenary session that took place in October 1996 in Bonn, Germany, brought together 187 delegates representing 39 member countries (among them the EU member states), and 19 international organizations. Two working parties were formed, one led by France on the values of nutritional references in labeling, the other led by the United States on methods of analysis.

There was a long debate on a different way of defining food information in general, and vitamins and minerals. There is currently no consensus on the negative and positive list system, and it will continue to be a major issue at the next plenary session, which is due to take place in September 1998.

The *Codex* applies to labeling and to claims relating to foodstuffs with special medical targets and that are in a category of dietary products especially formulated for dietary treatment of patients, and are specifically presented as such, and that cannot be used without medical advice.

These products can be taken exclusively or with other foods by patients with absorption or metabolic problems, or special dietary needs.

The labeling will include nutritional facts, minimal durability and the warning "only to be taken under medical supervision."

CONCLUSION

As I indicated at the start of this document, harmonization is achieved slowly, and we are today awaiting a report on the human diet from the CSAH, which is based in Brussels. The report, after consultation with the different member states, should lead to the establishment of a new community directive.

APPENDIX A

Decree 91-827 of 29-8-91

Food intended for a specific dietary requirement

1. *Foods for newborn babies*

2. *Milk and foods for babies*

3. *Foods for babies*

4. *Foods with low caloric value for weight control*

5. *Dietary foods for specific medical requirements*

6. *Foods low in sodium*

7. *Foods with no gluten*

8. *Foods for strong muscular efforts, mainly in sports*

9. *Foods for diabetic patients*

GLOSSARY

C.S.A.H.	*Comité Scientifique de l'Alimentation Humaine de l'Union Européenne (European Community Scientific Commitee for Foods)*
T.I.P.S.	*French for « Interministerial Tariff for Health Benefits »*
C.E.D.A.P.	*French for « Interministerial Commission on Products for a Special Diet »*
H.A.D.	*French for « Home Hospitalization »*

MEDICAL FOODS, THE UNITED STATES CONGRESS, AND THE FOOD AND DRUG ADMINSTRATION: A LOBBYING PRIMER AND COMMENTARY

Antonio C. Martinez II, Esq.
Calello Martinez PC
Nutley, NJ and Washington,DC

On November 29, 1996, the U.S. Food and Drug Administration published an Advanced Notice of Proposed Rulemaking on the Regulation of Medical Foods.[1] While industry and consumer interest in the area of medical foods has grown, it is critical to emphasize that interested parties must engage the agency and the U.S. Congress. Comments on the FDA proposal concluded on February 27, 1997. If left to its own devices, the FDA will ultimately propose a regulatory framework that both industry and consumers may not agree with. The FDA attempted to do this with the regulation of dietary supplements in the early 1990's and was rebuffed with the overwhelming passage of the Dietary Supplement Health and Education Act of 1994 (Public Law 103-417). All interested parties should begin the process of lobbying the Congress now. Lobbying simply defined is the education and advocacy of a particular public policy before the legislature. The bottom line is that Congress knows little about medical foods and what they have offer to our society and the economy.

[1]Federal Register Vol. 61, Number 231, pages 60661-60671

Industry and consumers are both left with a challenge: Does the current definition of Medical foods make sense? How should Medical Foods be regulated? What changes from your perspective would you like to see enacted? Congress has the power to clarify these uncertainties.

Bear in mind that there is a love-hate relationship with respect to Congress and the FDA. Congress always wants the FDA to be more efficient and more responsive. At the same time, it does not want to be perceived as weakening public health protection. This is the continual policy dance that both parties engage in. The FDA generally responds only to congressional pressures. If you depend solely upon the agency to take action, you may not be pleased with the result. As a rule of thumb, it is better to be proactive in developing public policy than reactive. Get the Congress involved.

The good news is that Congress is headed for major policy debates that open the door for discussion with medical foods. This includes:

1) the promotion and development of medical foods to respond to greater consumer and public health demand for such products.

2) the role of medical foods in managed health care plans.

3) the role of medical foods in Medicare. Do medical foods save health care dollars?

4) What is the level of science and technology available on medical foods?

5) Is the FDA a "user-friendly" agency in response to medical foods?

6) What are the actual problems with medical food regulations?

7) What improvements can be made at FDA with respect to medical foods?

HOW DO I START?

In the United States Congress, the Senate Committee of primary jurisdiction over health care policy is the Senate Labor and Human Resources Committee. The current makeup of the committee in the 105th Congress is eighteen members. The House Committee of primary jurisdiction over health care policy is the House Commerce Committee and its Subcommittee on Health and the Environment. The Commerce Committee has fifty-one members. In total, there are sixty nine men and women who directly affect any legislation that would concern Medical Foods. They are listed here for your convenience. These are the individuals who need to be educated and persuaded about medical foods.

ONE HUNDRED FIFTH CONGRESS

House Commerce Committee

(Ratio: 28-23)

Republicans
TOM BLILEY, VA, **CHAIRMAN**
W.J. "BILLY" TAUZIN, LA
MICHAEL G. OXLEY, OH
MICHAEL BILIRAKIS, FL
DAN SCHAEFER, CO
JOE BARTON, TX
J. DENNIS HASTERT, IL
FRED UPTON, MI
CLIFF STEARNS, FL
BILL PAXON, NY
PAUL E. GILLMOR, OH

SCOTT L. KLUG, WI
JAMES C. GREENWOOD, PA
MICHAEL D. CRAPO, ID
CHRISTOPHER COX, CA
NATHAN DEAL, GA
STEVE LARGENT, OK
RICHARD BURR, NC
BRIAN P. BILBRAY, CA
ED WHITFIELD, KY
GREG GANSKE, IA
CHARLIE NORWOOD, GA
RICK WHITE, WA
TOM COBURN, OK
RICK LAZIO, NY
BARBARA CUBIN, WY
JAMES ROGAN, CA
JOHN SHIMKUS, IL

Democrats
JOHN D. DINGELL, MI
HENRY A. WAXMAN, CA
EDWARD J. MARKEY, MA
RALPH M. HALL, TX
RICK BOUCHER, VA
THOMAS J. MANTON, NY
EDOLPHUS TOWNS NY
FRANK PALLONE JR., NJ
SHERROD BROWN, OH
BART GORDON, TN
ELIZABETH FURSE, OR
PETER DEUTSCH, FL
BOBBY L. RUSH, IL
ANNA G. ESHOO, CA
RON KLINK, PA
BART STUPAK, MI
ELIOT L. ENGEL, NY
THOMAS C. SAWYER, OH
ALBERT R. WYNN, MD
GENE GREEN, TX
KAREN MCCARTHY, MO
TED STRICKLAND, OH
DIANA DEGETTE, CO

Senate Committee on Labor and Human Resources
105th Congress
Ratio 10-8

REPUBLICANS:
JAMES JEFFORDS, VT **CHAIRMAN**
DAN COATS, IND
JUDD GREGG, NH
WILLIAM FRIST, TENN
MIKE DEWINE, OHIO
MIKE ENZI, WYO
TIM HUTCHINSON, ARK
SUSAN COLLINS, MAINE
JOHN WARNER, VA
MITCH MCCONNELL, KY

DEMOCRATS:
EDWARD KENNEDY, RANKING, MASS
CHRISTOPHER DODD, CONN
TOM HARKIN, IOWA
BARBARA MIKULSKI, MD
JEFF BINGAMAN, NM
PAUL WELLSTONE, MINN
PATTY MURRAY, WASH
JACK REED, R I

The upcoming debate on Medical Food regulation promises to be an interesting one. Hopefully, it will be a debate that you will choose not to sit idle and watch from the sidelines but become a major participant.

SAW PALMETTO BERRY IN THE TREATMENT OF BENIGN PROSTATIC HYPERPLASIA

Franklin C. Lowe, M.D., MPH, FACS

Departments of Urology, St. Lukes/Roosevelt

Hospital and Columbia University College of

Physicians and Surgeons

New York, NY 10019

ABSTRACT

Phytotherapeutic agents are widely used for treating the symptoms of benign prostatic hyperplasia (BPH). Saw palmetto berry (SPB) is the most widely studied of these agents. It's mechanism of action is poorly understood. It does not have 5-alpha-reductase activity. The active ingredient in this extract is also unknown.

There is much controversy concerning the efficacy of SPB. The double-blind trials, although usually favorable, do not show usual placebo response as seen in other BPH studies. Because of the variability of the natural history of BPH, the uncontrolled studies of these agents contribute little to determine efficacy. Further well-design placebo-controlled trials are necessary to establish the safety and efficacy of phytotherapy in the treatment of BPH.

INTRODUCTION

Phytotherapy, the use of plants or plant extracts for medicinal uses, has been described since ancient times, [1]as early as the 15th century BC in Egypt. The use of plants or plant extracts for the treatment of the symptoms of benign prostatic hyperplasia is widespread in Europe and gaining popularity in the United States.[2]

Other than the alpha-adrenergic blockers and hormonal agents (such as 5-alpha-reductase-inhibitors) which have Federal Drug Administration approval, most of the other phytotherapeutic, cholesterol-lowering agents, amino acid complexes or organ extracts have undergone little or no formal testing to determine efficacy in the treatment of prostatism. Saw palmetto berry extract (Serenoa repens) has undergone the most trials of any of these alternative therapies.

There are several difficulties in the evaluation of the effectiveness of phytotherapeutic agents for BPH. First, only a limited number of double-blind trials have been conducted; most studies have been uncontrolled. Results of uncontrolled studies should be regarded cautiously because a significant placebo effect of 40% - 60% has been observed in controlled studies of BPH. [3-6]Recent clinical trials with finasteride, terazosin and doxazosin have all demonstrated some moderate improvement with placebo.[7-9]Second, the active ingredient or ingredients of these agents are unknown. Therefore, the dosage of active medication being delivered by a specific preparation is also unknown, thus making comparison of similar medication from different manufacturers impossible. Third, in vitro experimental data regarding phytotherapeutic agents should be regarded cautiously because many of these studies use extremely high dosages of the extracts. Consequently, the levels of active ingredient or ingredients may be supraphysiologic and thus not relevant clinically. Finally, most previously reported clinical studies were not double-blind studies and did not utilize standardized symptom scores in their evaluation of treatment efficacy; thus, quantification and comparison of symptomatic improvement were not possible.

SAW PALMETTO BERRY

Saw palmetto is a dwarf palm tree of the family Arecaceae native to the West Indies and the South-Eastern United States. American Indians used saw palmetto berries for treatment of genitourinary disturbances and also as a nutritional tonic.[10] Saw palmetto was also believed to increase testicular function and relieve mucous membrane irritation.[10] The extract of the dried ripe fruit has been widely used for the treatment of BPH in Europe.[2],[1] Other common names for saw palmetto berry (SPB) include: dwarf palms, Serenoa repens, palmetto scrub, Sabal serrulata, or Sabalis serrulatae.[10] Numerous medications used for BPH contain SPB as one of their principal ingredients: Permixon(R), Curbicin(R), Prostaselect(R) and Strogen Forte(R).[1] SPB is found in combination in most prostate health pills sold in vitamin and health food stores.[2]

The lipid-soluble components of the saw palmetto berries are believed to contain the pharmacologically active components.[3] The purified lipid extract is used medicinally and consists of 85%-95% fatty acids and sterols. The steroid fraction is composed of beta-sitosterol, stigmasterol, cycloartenol, lupeol, lupenone, and methylcycloartenol.[10] Also present in the SBP extract are free fatty acids and long-chain alcohols. The pharmacologically active constituents are believed to be those compounds related to steroids; of these, sitosterols are believed to be the most important.[3] These compounds are chemically related to cholesterol, but their mechanism of action is still poorly understood.

EXPERIMENTAL DATA

The liposterolic extract of saw palmetto has been reported to possess antiandrogenic activity in vitro studies. Cell culture studies using human foreskin fibroblasts have demonstrated that the extract of saw palmetto competitively inhibits dihydrotestosterone (DHT) binding to both cytosolic and nuclear receptors.[11] Studies in rat prostate also show competitive inhibition of androgen binding to the cytosolic androgen receptor by saw palmetto berry extract.[12-14] In addition, inhibition of 5-alpha-reductase and 3-ketosteroid reductase (type 1) activity by extract of Serenoa repens has also been demonstrated in DU 145 cells, a metastatic human prostate carcinoma cell line.[15]

In contrast, studies by Rhodes et al.[16] have yielded conflicting results with those earlier studies. Permixon, an extract from Serenoa repens, did not demonstrate any inhibition of DHT binding to the rat prostatic androgen receptor. In addition, no evidence for inhibition of 5-alpha-reductase was seen. In castrated rats, Permixon was not able to inhibit testosterone-stimulated growth of the prostate; however, finasteride, a known 5-alpha-reductase inhibitor, did inhibit testosterone-stimulated growth in a dose-dependent manner.[16] Furthermore, in vitro studies using 5-alpha-reductase obtained from human prostate cells showed only minimal inhibitory activity of Permixon compared with finasteride.[16]

The results of Rhodes et al.[16] thus refute the theory that the action of saw palmetto is mediated through a 5-alpha-reductase inhibitory effect or through inhibition of androgen receptor binding. This clearly contradicts the results of Briley et al.[12],[13] and Carilla et al.[14] In all those studies, extremely high concentrations of Permixon (SPBE) were utilized; Rhodes et al. suggested that inhibition of 5-alpha-reductase and androgen binding is nonspecific at those high dosages. Furthermore, the dosages used by Carilla et al. and Briley et al. were supraphysiologic and thus are probably not clinically relevant. Clearly, further in vitro studies are necessary to determine the possible mechanism of action of saw palmetto.

CLINICAL STUDIES

Clinical studies in humans have not yielded any definitive data on the possible mechanism of action of saw palmetto. Casarosa et al.[17] treated 20 men with BPH with 320 mg of liposterolic extract of Serenoa repens for 1 month; no changes were seen in serum testosterone, follicle-stimulation hormone, or luteinizing hormone after 1 month of therapy. In addition, no evidence of 5-alpha-reductase inhibition has been demonstrated in clinical studies. Strauch et al.[18]treated 32 healthy male volunteers with 320 mg of Permixon for 1 week;

no change in serum DHT levels was seen. However, finasteride, 5 mg daily, was able to reduce DHT levels by 65%. These results have been confirmed by Rhodes et al.[16] in a separate experiment. In that study, 32 healthy men were treated with either 320 mg of Permixon, 5 mg of finasteride, or placebo for 1 week. Only the finasteride group showed any significant change, with an increase in serum testosterone and a decrease in serum DHT levels. Furthermore, there has been no demonstrable effect of SPB on serum prostate-specific antigen (PSA) levels; therefore, 5-alpha-reductase activity would be limited. Recent evaluation of 505 patients treated with 320 mg of SPB extract daily (Prostaserene) also showed no significant change in PSA levels.[19] Thus, SPB appears to have no 5-alpha-reductase activity.

Saw palmetto may affect steroid hormone receptor levels or activity after prolonged usage.[20] A double-blind study examined prostatic tissue obtained by suprapubic prostatectomy in 35 patients with BPH treated either with placebo or extract of Serenoa repens for 3 months.[20] The group treated with Serenoa repens showed a significant decrease in nuclear estrogen receptors and a decrease in nuclear androgen receptors in the prostate. Therefore, saw palmetto's effect might be medicated through alterations in androgen and estrogen action.

Overall, the mechanism of action of saw palmetto berry remains to be determined. Clinical studies suggest that there is no appreciable inhibition of 5-alpha-reductase or change in PSA levels. Furthermore, there have been conflicting reports on the inhibition of testosterone binding by SPB. Estrogen and androgen receptor levels may be affected by treatment; however, confirmation is needed. Clearly, further investigations will be needed to establish the effect, if any, of Serenoa repens on hormone metabolism in BPH.

CLINICAL TRIALS

Although several trials have been conducted on the effectiveness of

TABLE I. Double-blind placebo-controlled studies using saw palmetto berry extract for treatment of benign prostatic hyperplasia

STUDY	Year	Agent	Daily Dose (mg)	Total No. of Pts.	Study Duration (mo)	Symptoms	Change in flow Rate (cc/s) Treated	Placebo
Boccafoschi and Annoscia[22]	1983	Permixon	320	22	2	Decreased	4.1*	1.9
Emili et al[23]	1983	Permixon	320	30	1	Decreased	3.4*	0.2
Champault et al.[21]	1984	PA109	320	110	1	Decreased	3.0*	0.3
Cukier et al.[25]	1985	Permixon	320	146	2	Decreased	NA	NA
Tasca et al.[24]	1985	PA109	320	30	1-3	Decreased	3.3*	0.6
Reese Smith et al.[27]	1986	Permixon	320	70	3	Not Decreased	2.5	2.5
Carbin et al.[26]	1990	Curbicin	480	53	3	Decreased	3.0*	0.6

KEY; Pts = patients; NA + not available
*P <0.05 versus photo** Adapted from Lowe and Ku, Urology 48:14, 1996

phytotherapeutic drugs, the vast majority were short term and uncontrolled.[1-3] Only a limited number of double-blind, placebo-controlled studies on Serenoa repens have been reported (Table I).

Placebo Controlled Studies. Champault et al.[21] treated 110 patients in a double-blind, placebo-controlled study with extract of Serenoa repens (PA109). Patients were treated with 320 mg of PA109/day or placebo for 30 days. Statistically significant improvement in nocturia, dysuria, and overall assessment was seen in the treatment group versus the placebo group. In the treatment group, flow rate increased from 5.3 to 8.0 cc/s ($P < 0.001$); the placebo group showed no significant change in flow rate (before treatment, 5.0 cc/s; after treatment, 5.3 cc/s). The finding that the placebo-treated patients exhibited no improvement is in contradistinction to numerous pharmaceutical clinical studies that have all shown some improvement in the placebo groups.[7-9]

Boccafoschi and Annoscia,[21] in a double-blind trial of 22 patients treated with Permixon (320 mg daily) for 2 months, demonstrated a significant increase in flow rate and a decrease in PVR in the treatment group. Flow rate increased from 9.6 cc/s initially to 13.7 cc/s; residual urine decreased from 103 cc initially to 55 cc. In the placebo group, flow rate increased from 10.2 cc/s initially to 12.2 cc/s, and PVR decreased for 66 to 36 cc. This was the only double-blind study to show some improvement in the placebo control arm for both flow rate (1.9 cc/s) and PVR (29 cc).

A double-blind trial by Emili et al.[23] using Permixon (320 mg daily) for 1 month in 30 patients also showed a significant increase in flow rate and a decrease in PVR. Flow rate increased by 3.4 cc/s, and PVR decreased from an initial value of 71 to 36 cc. No appreciable change was seen in the placebo group. Tasca et al[24]also reported significant increase in flow rate after treatment with 320 mg of PA109 daily for 1 to 3 months in a double-blind study. Again, no significant change was seen in the placebo group, although a minor increase in flow rate (0.6 cc/s) was observed. Cukier et al.[28] in a double-blind study of 146 patients, reported a significant lessening of symptoms and a decrease in PVR after 2 months of treatment with Permixon.

Carbin et al.[26] treated 53 patients for 3 months in a double-blind, placebo-controlled study using the agent Curbicin, which is derived from Sabal serrulata and pumpkin seeds. Improvements in both flow rate (before treatment, 6.7 cc/s; after treatment 9.7 cc/s, $P < 0.001$) and PVR (before treatment, 135 cc; after treatment, 92 cc, $P < 0.01$) was seen in the treatment group. No significant change was observed in the placebo group. In addition, significant improvement in frequency, nocturia, dysuria, and overall assessment was seen in the treatment group.

In contrast, a double-blind study by Reese Smith et al.[27]showed no significant difference between saw palmetto (Permixon) and placebo. In that study, 80 patients were randomized to receive either Permixon (an extract of Serenoa repens, 320 mg/day) or placebo for 3 months; 70 patients were evaluable. Symptomatic improvement was seen in both groups, but no statistical difference between the individual groups was demonstrated. A significant increase in flow rates was seen in both groups (2.5 cc/s), but the difference between treated and placebo groups was not significant. The PVR values were variable and essentially unchanged for both groups. The study of Reese Smith et al. was the only critical double-blind study of SPB and showed the greatest effect of placebo-treated patients. This improvement was comparable to that seen in the placebo control arms of recent clinical trials of finasteride, doxazosin, and terazosin.[7-9]Thus, these data seem to be the most believable.

Uncontrolled Studies. Uncontrolled studies have also reported improvement in both objective and subjective variables.[19, 28-31] The largest uncontrolled study of 1334 patients treated with 160 mg of SPB extract (Talso) twice daily for 6 months was reported by Vahlensieck et al.[30]from Germany. It showed improvement in PVR (50% decrease), frequency (37% decrease) and nocturia (54% decrease); overall assessment was rated good to excellent by 80% of the patients.

Results of a multicenter open-label study in Belgium were recently reported.[19] In that trial, 505 patients were treated with Serenoa repens extract (320 mg/day) for 3 months. A significant decrease in prostate symptom scores (International Prostate Symptom Score [IPSS]) was demonstrated. At 45 days, a 22% decrease was documented; by 90 days, symptom scores were decreased by 35%. The absolute symptom scores were decreased from 19.0 to 12.4 ($P < 0.001$). In addition, the maximum flow rate increased for 9.8 to 12.2 cc/s ($P < 0.001$). Although an uncontrolled study, it was clearly the most rigorous and well constructed in that it measured prostate volume, PSA levels, and flow rates, in addition, IPSS symptom scores were utilized.

Finasteride Controlled Study. In a double-blind, multicenter, European comparison trial between Permixon and finasteride was undertaken to determine equivalency.[32] 1098 patients were randomized to either 320 mg of Permixon or 5 mg of finasteride. Primary outcome measurement was the International

Prostate Symptom Score. After six months of therapy, both arms of the trial showed improvement -37% with Permixon and -39% with finasteride.[32] Quality of Life and flow rates were also showed comparable improvements.

Premature withdrawal was 16% with Permixon and 11% with finasteride. Side effects causing premature withdrawal was twice as common for Permixon (28 versus 14 patients). The decreased libido and impotence incidences were 2.2% versus 3.0% and 1.5% versus 2.8 for Permixon and finasteride respectively.

Although this well designed and carried out trial supports the equivalency of Permixon to finasteride in treating men with moderate to severe symptoms of BPH; recent study by Dr. Lepor in the New England Journal of Medicine indicated that finasteride was not statistically better than placebo.[33] Therefore, comparing Permixon to finasteride might have simply showing equivalency to placebo.

SUMMARY OF CLINICAL STUDIES OF SPB

Overall, the studies evaluating the efficacy of SPB extract are inconclusive because of problems with inclusion/exclusion criteria, lack of uniform symptom score analysis, and very short duration of therapy (no more than 3 months). However, six of the seven double-blind studies showed improvement in both objective and subjective variables of BPH over only 1 to 3 months. The magnitude of the symptomatic improvement could not be quantitated because no standardized symptom score system was utilized. Additionally, only two of the seven studies showed any improvement with placebo therapy. For example, the 3-month trial by Reece Smith et al.[27] demonstrated a significant increase in flow rate and decrease in symptoms with both placebo and SPB; therefore, it was concluded that SPB was no better than placebo.

That these studies did not show any improvement in the placebo arms is in contradistinction to the placebo-controlled studies using various other BPH medications (terazosin, doxasosin, and finasteride), which have always shown some improvement with placebo.[4,6,7,8] In fact, the control arm of a terazosin study showed that 40% of the patients reported a greater that 30% decrease in symptom scores, and 25% had a greater than 30% increase in maximum flow rate.[8] Therefore, the controlled studies cited here that showed improvement with SPB extract treatment should be regarded cautiously.

The uncontrolled studies all showed favorable results with the usage of SPB extract; however, without a control arm, these data are all questionable because of the variability of the natural history of BPH. For example, Ball et al.[34] observed 97 patients with prostatism with therapy for 5 years. Ten patients required surgery for worsening symptoms; however, 31 patients reported lessened symptoms after observation alone, and 50 reported no change. Thus, the uncontrolled studies with SPB extract are not useful in defining the legitimate role of this agent in the treatment of BPH.[37]

SUMMARY

Phytotherapeutic agents have enjoyed widespread use, especially in Europe, for the treatment of BPH. With the recent proliferation of nutrition and vitamin stores in the United States, use of these agents has greatly increased.[2] Although SPB extract is the most extensively studied of the phytotherapeutic agents used for BPH, no well-defined mechanism of action has been proposed. Evidence for an antiandrogenic or antiestrogenic effect is conflicting, and there are no clinical data suggesting an effect on 5-alpha-reductase activity. Furthermore, clinical trials with SPB have largely been uncontrolled and are thus of limited value in ascertaining the true clinical impact of this agent. Double-blind, controlled studies with SPB also have limitations in that most were of very short duration (none longer than 3 months) and did not provide entry or exclusion criteria. In addition, standardized symptom scores were not utilized. Only two of seven studies showed an appropriate placebo response, and the results and conclusions of both of these studies were contradictory.[22,27]

The best and most convincing study of the efficacy of phytotherapeutic agents (using Harzol, a combination of beta-sitosterols) was recently published in the Lancet.[35] This study was rigorous and matched in design and format with pharmaceutical industry trials. A mild but appropriate placebo response was detected, which further validates the study. However, a prior placebo-controlled study showed no efficacy of betasitosterol-beta-D-glucoside.[36] This dichotomy of results possibly reflects the different composition of the agents tested. This is a major confounding factor in this field of study, especially because the active ingredients are unknown. Standardization of the compounds is needed to compare and assess accurately the effect of the different extracts.[37]

CONCLUSIONS

The evidence for the efficacy of phytotherapeutic agents in the treatment of symptomatic BPH is inconclusive.[37] Unless other appropriate studies and trials are conducted to confirm their efficacy, it is difficult to refute the belief that these phytotherapeutic agents are no more than an expensive form of placebo.

Because many of the medicines used in clinical practice are derived from the plant world, it is conceivable that these agents do have some benefit for the treatment of BPH. The widespread usage and demand for these agents certainly warrant further well-designed, longer-term placebo-controlled studies.[37]

REFERENCES

1. Dreikorn K, and Richter R: Conservative nonhormonal treatment of patients with benign prostatic hyperplasia, in Ackerman R, and Schroeder FH (Eds): *New Developments in Biosciences 5, Prostatic Hyperplasia*. Berlin, New York, Walter de Gruyter & Co., 1989, pp 109-131.

2. Marwick C: Growing use of medicinal botanicals forces assessment by drug regulators. JAMA 273: 607-609, 1995.

3. Di Silverio F, Flammia GP, Sciarra A, Caponera M, Mauro M, Buscarini M, Tavani M, and D, Eramo G: Plant extracts in BPH. Minerva Urol Nefrol 45: 143-149, 1993.

4. Wein AJ: Assessing treatment results in benign prostatic hyperplasia. Urol Clin North Am 22:345-355, 1995.

5. Barry MJ, Girman CJ, O'Leary MP, Walker-Corkery Prostatic Hyperplasia Treatment Outcomes Study Group: Using repeated measures of symptom score, uroflowmetry, and prostate specific antigen in the clinical management of prostate disease.

6. Schulze H, Berges R, Paschold K, and Senge T: Neue konservative therapieausaetze bei der benignen prostahyperplasie. Urologe A 31:8-13, 1982.

7. Gormley GJ, Stoner, Bruskewitz RC, and the Finasteride Study Group: The effect of finasteride in men with benign prostatic hyperplasia. N Engl J Med 327: 1185-1191,1992.

8. Lepor H: Alpha blockade for the treatment of benign prostatic hyperplasia. Urol Clin North Am 22: 375-386, 1995.

9. Gillenwater JY, and Mobley DL: A sixteen week, double-blind, placebo-controlled, dose-titration study using doxazosin tablets for the treatment of benign prostatic hyperplasia (BPH) in normotensive males: a multicenter study group (abstract). J Urol 149: 324A, 1993.

10. Murray M, and Pizzorno J: *Encyclopedia of Natural Medicine*. Seattle, John Bastyr University Publishing, 1994.

11. Sultan C, Terraza A, Devillier C, Carilla E, Briley M, Loire C, and Descomps B: Inhibition of androgen metabolism and binding by a liposterolic extract of :serenoa repens B" in human foreskin fibroblasts. J Steroid Biochem 20: 515-519, 1984.

12. Briley M, Carilla E, and Roger A: Inhibitory effect of Permixon on testosterone 5 alpha reductase activity of the rat ventral prostate. Br J Pharmacol 83:401P, 1984.

13.Briley M, Carilla E, and Fauran F: Permixon, a new treatment for benign prostatic hyperplasia, acts directly at the cytosolic androgen receptor in rat prostate. Br J Pharmacol 79: 327P, 1983.

14. Carilla E, Briley M, Fauran F, Sultan C, and Duvilliers C: Binding of Permixon, a new treatment for prostatic benign hyperplasia, to the cytosolic androgen receptor in the rat prostate. J Steroid Biochem 20: 521-523, 1984.

15. Delos S, Iehle C, Martin PM, and Raynaud JP: Inhibition of the activity of 'basic' 5 alpha reductase (type 1) detected in DU 145 cells and expressed in insect cells. J Steroid Biochem 48: 347-352, 1994.

16. Rhodes L, Primka RL, Berman C, Vergult G, Gabriel M, Pierre-Malice M, and Gibelin B: Comparison of finasteride (Proscar), a 5 alpha reductase inhibitor, and various commercial plant extracts in vitro and in vivo 5 alpha reductase inhibition. Prostate 22: 43-51, 1993.

17. Casarosa C, diCoscio MC, and Fratta M: Lack of effects of a lyposterolic extract of Serenoa repens on plasma levels of testosterone, follicle-stimulating hormone, and luteinizing hormone. Clin Ther 10:585-588, 1988.

18. Strauch G, Perles P, Vergult G, Gabriel M, Gibelin B, Cummings S, Malbecq W, and Malice MP: Comparison of finasteride (Proscar) and Serenoa repens (Permixon) in the inhibition of 5 alpha reductase in healthy male volunteers Eur Urol 26: 247-252, 1994.

19. Braeckman J: The extract of Serenoa repens in the treatment of benign prostatic hyperplasia: a multicenter open study. Curr Ther Res 55: 776, 1994.

20. Di Silverio F, D'Eramo G, Lubrano C, Flammia GP Sciarra A, Palma E, Caponera M, and Sciarra F: Evidence that Serenoa repens extract displays and antiestogenic activity in prostatic tissue of benign prostatic hypertrophy patients. Eur Urol 21: 309-314, 1992.

21. Champault G, Patel JC, and Bonnard AML A double-blind trial of an extract of the plant Serenoa repens in benign prostatic hyperplasia. Br J Clin Pharmacol 18: 461-462, 1984.

22. Boccafoschi C, and Annoscia S: Confronto fra estratto di serenoa repens e placebo mediate proba clinica controllata in pazienti con adenomatosi prostatica. Urologia 50: 1257-1268, 1983.

23. Emili E, Lo Cign M, and Petrone U: Risultati clinici su un nuovo farmaco nella terapia dell'ipertrofia della prostata (Permixon). Urologia 50: 1042-1048, 1983.

24. Tasca A, Barulla M, Cavazzana A, Zattoni F, Artibani W, and Pagano F: Trattamento della sintomatologia ostruttiva de adenoma prostatico conestratto di Serenoa Repens. Minerva Urol Nefro 37: 87-91, 1985.

25. Cukier P, Ducassou P, Le Guillou P, Leriche P, Lobel P, Toubol P, coremieux D, Frinenwald D, Pastorini D, Raymond D, Reziciner C, And Martinaggi D: Permixon versus placebo; Resultats d'une etude multicentrique. C R Ther Pharmacol Clin 4: 15-21, 1985.

26. Carbin BE, Larsson B, and Lindahl O: Treatment of benign prostatic hyperplasia with phytosterols. Br J Urol 66: 629-641, 1990.

27. Reese Smith H, Memon A, Smart CJ, and Dewbury K: The value of permixon in benign prostatic hypertrophy. Br J Jurol 58: 36-40, 1986.

28. Di Silverio F, D'Eramo G, Flammis GP, Buscarini M, Reascaro E, Mariani M, and Sciarra A: Associations pharmacologiques dans le tritement de l'hypertrophie prostatique benigne. J Urol 99: 316-320, 1993.

29. Romics I, Schmitz H, and Frang D: Experience in treating benign prostatic hypertrophy with Sabal serrulata for one year. Int Urol Nephrol 25: 565-569, 1993.

30. Vahlensieck W Jr, Volp A, Lubos W, and Kuntze M; Benigne prostatahyperplasie-benhandlung mit sabalfrucht-estrakt. Fortschr Med 111: 323-326, 1993.

31. Cirillio-Marucco, Pagliarula A, Trito G, Piccinno A, and EiRienzo U: L'estratto di serenoa repens (Permixon) nel trattamento precoce dell'ipertrofia prostatica. Urologia 50: 1269-1277, 1983.

32. DiSilverio, F ad the Permixon Study Group: Comparison of Phytotherapy (Permixon) with Finasteride in the Treatment of Benign Prostatic Hyperplasia: A Randomized International Study of 1098 Patients. J. Urol. 155:576A, 1996.

33. Lepor, H, Williford, WO, Barry, MJ et al: The efficacy of terazosin, finasteride, or both in benign prostatic hyperplasia. N. Engl. J Med. 335:533-539, 1996.

34. Ball AJ, Feneley RC, and Abrams PH: The natural history of untreated "prostatism." Br J Urol 53: 613-616, 1981.

35. Berges RR, Windeler J, Trampisch HJ, Senge T, and the Beta-Sitosterol Study Group: Randomised, placebo-controlled, double-blind clinical trial of beta-sitosterol in patients with benign prostatic hyperplasia. Lancet 345: 1529-1532, 1995.

36. Kadow C, and Abrams PH: A double-blind trial of the effect of beta-sitosteryl glucoside (WA184) in the treatment of benign prostatic hyperplasia. Eur Urol 12:187-189, 1986.

37. Lowe, FC and KU, JC: Phytotherapy in the Treatment of Benign Prostatic Hyperplasia: A Critical Review Urology 48: 12-20, 1996.

CARDIA SALT ALTERNATIVE

Fredric Price
President & CEO
Applied Microbiology, Inc
Tarrytown, NY

What is Cardia Salt Alternative, how does it work, and what makes it different from other salts?

Cardia Salt Alternative looks, cooks, and tastes just like salt. In addition to its dietary blood pressure-lowering effects, published pre-clinical data show it did not interfere with the leading antihypertensive drugs such as ACE-inhibitors and beta-blockers. Studies have shown that regular salt does interfere with the blood pressure-lowering effects of these medications; this interference can lead to additional physician visits, as well as to adjustments in medication section and dosing, which can result in increased healthcare costs and lower quality of life for hypertensive patients. Cardia Salt Alternative provides an opportunity for hypertensive patients to enjoy the good taste of salt—guilt-free—while enabling them to comply with the recommendations of their physicians, pharmacists, and dietitians to reduce sodium and maintain the essential minerals potassium and magnesium in their daily diets.

This paper has been presented elsewhere.

Cardia's unique formulation—including 54% less sodium than regular salt plus the important minerals potassium and magnesium—and good salt taste resulted in the issuance of a US composition-of-matter patent.

Cardia Salt Alternative is unique for the following reasons:

- Published clinical (double-blind, placebo-controlled) studies have shown that Cardia Salt Alternative reduces blood pressure when included in the diet in place of regular salt

- Published preclinical data indicate that Cardia Salt Alternative does not interfere with the effects of antihypertensive agents, unlike regular salt

- Double-blind, placebo-controlled taste tests demonstrate that Cardia Salt Alternative delivers the same salty taste as table salt

- It complies with the recommendations of the National Heart, Lung and Blood Institute (NHLBI) regarding lifestyle modifications for hypertension control and/or overall cardiovascular risk

- It complies with the recommendations of the Expert Panel on the role of dietary sodium and potassium in the prevention and management of hypertension

Why is it important to replace regular salt with Cardia Salt Alternative?

An estimated 50 million Americans have high blood pressure and a significant percentage of them continue to use salt (sodium chloride) in their diets. Numerous epidemiological and clinical studies have shown that diets low in sodium and high in potassium help prevent and manage high blood pressure.

The NHLBI and the American Heart Association (AHA) recommend that Americans reduce their salt intake to 6 grams per day (2.3 grams of sodium) and maintain adequate dietary potassium. Despite these guidelines, on average, Americans continue to consume twice the recommended daily intake of sodium and insufficient amounts of potassium.

In fact, it is estimated that adult Americans consume more than 900,000,000 pounds of excess salt each year, which can not only increase the risk of developing hypertension but also can interfere with the therapeutic effects of most antihypertensive drugs. Recently, a panel of leading experts in hypertension was convened in New York City on December 5, 1996 under the auspices of the Columbia University School of Public Health to consider current data on the role of dietary sodium, potassium and other minerals in the prevention and management of hypertension. During the course of individual presentations and discussion, the panel reached consensus on several important issues and their implications for people with normal blood pressure and for people with hypertension.

Is there a relationship between sodium and high blood pressure?

Significant clinical evidence exists to support a causal relationship between sodium (salt) consumption and high blood pressure. Some of the clinical data presented by conference participants indicate that restricting salt consumption can be an effective alternative to the use of diuretic medicines for some people with high blood pressure. Data also show that reducing dietary sodium may enhance the effect of antihypertensive drugs, especially beta-blockers, diuretics and ACE inhibitors.

Who benefits from reducing the amount of salt in the diet?

The panel agreed that all people would benefit from moderating their daily sodium intake while focusing on eating potassium-rich foods. People with high blood pressure who are already taking blood pressure medicines may experience a further blood pressure reduction if they limit dietary salt, but the degree of benefit can vary from patient to patient depending on the medicines they are taking and their sensitivity to sodium. Certain sub-populations are more sensitive than others to the effects of sodium. Salt restriction is of critical importance for these people, but the Panel felt that all Americans should be careful about salt intake to help avoid the onset of high blood pressure.

Is there a relationship between potassium or magnesium deficiency and hypertension?

The panel agreed that all people would benefit by adhering to the recommendations of the National High Blood Pressure Education Program to maintain adequate dietary intake of calcium, potassium and magnesium. There is a correlation between low potassium intake and a higher incidence of hypertension and cardiovascular disease. Clinical and epidemiological studies have demonstrated that potassium supplementation may be quite effective in reducing blood pressure, especially in people who cannot or will not reduce sodium intake. There are some data on the effect of magnesium deficiency on blood pressure, but the data are equivocal and more study is required.

Effective implementation of these recommendations would result in significantly less deaths from strokes and heart attacks. According to a published study,

(Law et al., (1991) BMJ, 302;811-824 Meta-analysis of 47,000 subjects), the reduction of salt intake of 3 grams per day would result in an annual decrease in deaths from stroke by 22% and heart attack by 16%; while a reduction of salt intake of 6 grams per day would result in annual decreases of each cardiovascular event by 39% and 30% respectively. Despite intense efforts to disseminate the message that excess sodium can contribute to high blood pressure, sodium intake for the average American adult is twice the recommendations of the NHLBI and the AHA, as people have come to enjoy the taste of regular salt.

Have any clinical studies been presented recently supporting the recommendations for reduced sodium intake for hypertensive patients?

Joel, Neutel MD, Director, Hypertension and Cardiovascular Research, Orange County Heart Institute, presented the clinical data describing the benefits of Cardia Salt Alternative on blood pressure at the 69th Scientific Session of the American Heart Association held in November 1996 and published in a supplement of Circulation, 1996, Volume 94, No. 8, Page 1983. Included in his presentation were the results of a six month study of 40 mild to moderate hypertensive patients who were placed on salt restricted diets and randomized to receive either Cardia Salt Alternative or regular salt. In the Cardia Salt Alternative Group, both systolic and diastolic blood pressure were reduced in a statistically significant manner by 13 and 8 millimeters of mercury respectively. A non-significant reduction in systolic and diastolic blood pressure of 8 and 5 millimeters of mercury was also observed in the regular salt group; an effect that was attributed to a reduction in sodium intake by itself.

What are the recommended lifestyle modifications for people with high blood pressure?

The National Institutes of Health issued a report from their Joint National Committee on the Detection, Evaluation, and Treatment of High Blood Pressure (JNC-V) in 1993 which recommended several lifestyle modifications for hypertension control and/or overall cardiovascular risk. These recommendations include:

- Lose weight if overweight.

- Limit alcohol intake to no more than 1 ounce of ethanol per day (24 ounces of beer, 8 ounces of wine, or 2 ounces of 100 proof whiskey).

- Exercise (aerobic) regularly.

- Reduce sodium intake to less than 100 mmol (<2.3 grams of sodium or < 6 grams of sodium chloride).

- Maintain adequate dietary potassium, calcium, and magnesium intake.

- Stop smoking and reduce dietary fat and cholesterol intake for overall cardiovascular health. Reducing fat intake also helps reduce caloric intake – important for control of weight and Type II diabetes.

How and to whom is Cardia Salt Alternative marketed?

Cardia Salt Alternative was launched in the US in test markets in April 1996. In January 1997, the product was launched nationally and is currently available in pharmacies throughout the US. Cardia Salt Alternative is being marketed to patients with high blood pressure who cannot give up the taste of salt. The Company has developed marketing programs for physicians, pharmacists, and dietitians to recommend the product for those patients with high blood pressure. These programs are designed to create product awareness, stimulate trial usage, and expand recommendations from health care professionals.

Zbar as a Part of the Diabetes Regimen

Francine Ratner Kaufman, M.D.
Associate Professor of Pediatrics
University of Southern California School of Medicine
Director, Comprehensive Childhood Diabetes Program
Childrens Hospital Los Angeles

The Department of Pediatrics, Childrens Hospital Los Angeles and the University of Southern California School of Medicine, Los Angeles, California

INTRODUCTION

We first reported on the benefit of uncooked cornstarch, as an adjunct to the diabetes regimen, in 1994, after the Diabetes Control and Complication Trial (1993) (1) unequivocally demonstrated that meticulous glycemic control resulted in a marked decrease in the incidence and progression of the chronic complications of type 1 diabetes mellitus. As a large urban center caring for a diverse type 1 pediatric diabetes population, we had already begun to see an increase in severe hypoglycemia in our patients as we intensified diabetes management. Since we had already been using large quantities of uncooked cornstarch to successfully diminish the hypoglycemia seen in other patients with glycogen storage diseases (2) and other hypoglycemic syndromes, we began to investigate whether there was a role for uncooked cornstarch in diabetes.

Uncooked cornstarch is a complex carbohydrate composed of approximately 73% of the branched chain dextrose polymer, amylopectin, and 27% of the linear chain dextrose polymer, amylose. Uncooked cornstarch requires pancreatic amylase for hydrolysis. This process appears to occur slowly in the gastrointestinal tract, allowing for the extended absorption of liberated monosaccharides into the systemic circulation over hours. Through this mechanism, in addition to perhaps others, it appears that uncooked cornstarch can help prolong the post-absorptive state to diminish the risk of hypoglycemia for up to 6-7 hours. This paper reports on our initial studies using uncooked cornstarch as part of the evening snack in subjects with diabetes. These initial investigations led to the formulation of Zbar and its evaluation in children with this chronic disease.

RESEARCH STUDIES

In 1994, we began our pilot study (3) to determine if uncooked cornstarch, combined with other complex carbohydrate, fat and protein, to be ingested as the evening snack could be used to diminish the nocturnal hypoglycemia seen in intensively managed children with diabetes. Thirteen children and adolescents were recruited into this study after they signed an informed consent. These subjects adhered to an intensive diabetes management protocol involving two to three insulin injections per day or using a closed-loop subcutaneous insulin infusion pump. They had a mean HbA1C of 6.8 ± 0.7%, indicating that they had achieved the level of glycemic control advocated by the Diabetes Control and Complication Trial (1). The study protocol compared blood glucose levels at 0200 and 0700 for four weeks; two weeks during which time a standard predetermined evening snack was ingested, followed by a two week period in which the evening snack contained 5-7 grams of uncooked cornstarch. The mean glucose levels at 0700 and the number of hypoglycemic episodes, as defined as a blood glucose by finger stick of < 60 mg/dL, at 0200 and 0700 are given in Table 1. There was no difference in mean fasting blood glucose levels in the morning, however, there was a decrease in the mean number of hypoglycemic episodes at 0200 and 0700 during the time period in which the cornstarch snack was ingested compared to the standard snack.

Table 1. Comparison of Mean Fasting Blood Glucose Levels and Episodes of Hypoglycemia with a Standard Snack Compared to a Cornstarch Snack in Thirteen Children Following an Intensive Management Protocol

	Mean Fasting Glucose	Mean Number Hypoglycemic Episodes	
	0700	0200	0700
Standard Snack	138 ± 38 mg/dL	2.00 ± 2.12	2.61 ± 2.25
Cornstarch Snack	143 ± 30 mg/dL	0.61 ± 0.87	0.69 ± 1.03
	$p>0.10$	$p<0.025$	$p<0.01$

Four children had glucose levels every two hours through the night after cornstarch ingestion and they achieved stable glycemia without the development of hypoglycemia. These data were highly suggestive that a small amount of uncooked cornstarch added to the evening snack of children with intensively managed diabetes resulted in a reduction in hypoglycemic episodes without inducing hyperglycemia.

The next study that was conducted expanded on the number of subjects evaluated and was conducted at diabetes camp (4). Fifty one campers and counselors at the American Diabetes Association sponsored summer camp in the San Bernardino

Mountains of Southern California entered this study after they signed an informed consent. Study participants were randomized to receive 5 nights of a standard snack and 5 nights of a snack in which 5 grams of carbohydrate was replaced with uncooked cornstarch. Participants and medical personnel were masked as to which snacks were given. Midnight and 0700 finger stick blood glucose levels were compared with values < 60 mg/dL defined as hypoglycemia and values > 250 mg/dL defined as hyperglycemia.

Comparisons were made for 218 midnight and 222 morning glucose values. Results of this study, which are shown in Table 2, revealed that there was a significant decrease in hypoglycemia at midnight and in the morning with no increase in hyperglycemia when the cornstarch snack was ingested compared to the standard snack. In addition, the number of campers to ever experience hypoglycemia (12% with the cornstarch snack compared to 46% with the standard snack at midnight, $p<0.001$; 16% with the cornstarch snack compared to 26% with the standard snack at 0700, $p=0.327$) was reduced with the addition of cornstarch.

This study revealed that cornstarch could have benefit in a wider range of subjects who had more variability in their overall diabetes control. However, the campers and counselors informed us at the completion of this study that the snacks were not tasty and that they would not routinely use uncooked cornstarch because it was not convenient or palatable. This led to the formulation of Zbar in an attempt to find a premeasured, easy to use and tasty product that would have appeal to a wide range of subjects with diabetes. The formulation that resulted in Zbar is given in Table 3.

During the following summer of 1995, another trial was conducted at diabetes camp comparing Zbar to a Placebo Bar of equal calories and nutrient content but

Table 2. Comparison of Hypoglycemic and Hyperglycemic Events with the Cornstarch Snack compared to the Standard Snack in 51 Campers

	Morning	Midnight
HYPOGLYCEMIC EVENTS		
Standard Snack	21	30
Cornstarch Snack	9	6
	$p<0.05$	$p<0.001$
HYPERGLYCEMIC EVENTS		
Standard Snack	19	23
Cornstarch Snack	26	13
	$p=0.273$	$p=0.112$

without uncooked cornstarch (5). For this study, 79 adolescent campers and counselors were randomally assigned to Group A (5 nights of the Zbar, followed by 5 nights of Placebo Bar) or Group B (5 nights of Placebo Bar followed by 5 nights of Zbar) after they signed informed consent. Again, counselors, campers and medical personnel were blinded as to snack bar assignment. Hypoglycemic and hyperglycemic episodes were analyzed for the total cohort, by Group assignment and by glycated hemoglobin quartiles. As shown in Figure 1, there was a significant reduction in the number of hypoglycemic events with Zbar

Table 3. Composition of Cornstarch Bar

Nutrition Facts
Serving Size 1 Bar (33 g/1.2 oz)

Amount Per Serving		% Daily Value based on 2000 Calories	DRV for 2000 Calories
Calories	110		
Calories from Fat	25		
Total Fat	2.5 g	4%	65 g
Saturated Fat	0 g	0%	20 g
Monounsaturated Fat	1 g		
Polyunsaturated Fat	1 g		
Cholesterol	0 mg	0	300 mg
Sodium	90 mg	4%	2400 mg
Potassium	90 mg	3%	3500 mg
Total Carbohydrate	22 mg	7%	300 g
Dietary Fiber	1 g	4%	25 g
Sugars	1 g		
Sugar Alcohol	8 g		
Other Carbohydrate*			
Protein	7 g		

Vitamin A	**	Folate	2%
Vitamin C	**	Vitamin B12	**
Calcium	4%	Biotin	**
Iron	4%	Pantothenic	**
Vitamin D	**	Phosphorus	8%
Vitamin E	**	Iodine	2%
Thiamin	**	Magnesium	4%
Riboflavin	2%	Zinc	2%
Niacin	**	Copper	4%
Vitamin B6	**		

* Cornstarch 5 grams

compared to the Placebo Bar at midnight and in the morning and a significant decrease in the number of subjects to ever experience hypoglycemia with Zbar compared to the Placebo Bar. These differences held across the glycated hemoglobin quartiles, therefore, the hypoglycemic protective effect of Zbar was independent of antecedent diabetes control.

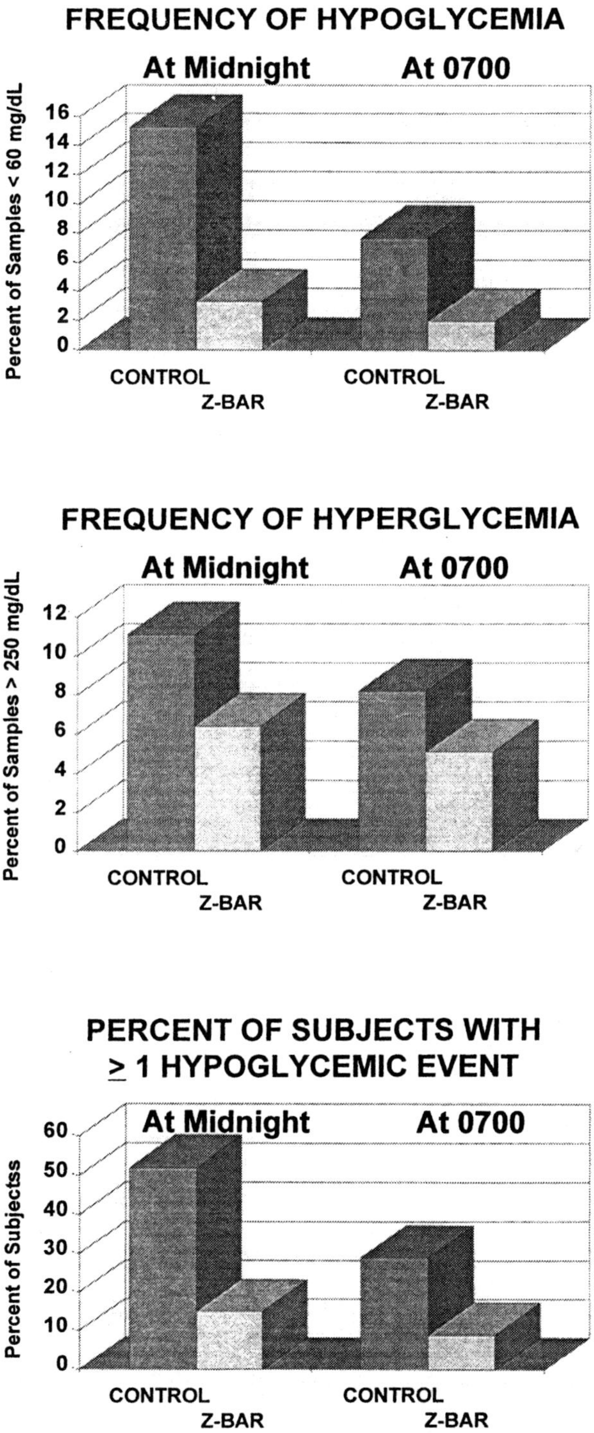

Figure 1 Frequency of Hypoglycemia, Hyperglycemic and Percent of Subjects with ≥ 1 Hypoglycemic Events with Zbar vs Control Bar

More importantly, after the code was broken, the subjects stated that Zbar was tasty and easy to incorporate in their meal plans. The teens and young adults who had entered this study felt that Zbar was an adequate snack when combined with fluid (non- or low-fat milk) and that they did not experience hunger after ingestion of Zbar as the evening snack. They felt that with the significant reduction of hypoglycemia in the middle of the night and in the morning, without increasing hyperglycemia, Zbar would be of great value as an adjunct in diabetes management to improve long term outcome.

REFERENCES

1. The Diabetes Control and Complication Trial. The effect of intensive diabetes management on the development and progression of long-term complications in insulin dependent diabetes mellitus: the diabetes control and complication trial. N Engl J Med 1993;329:977-987.

2. Chen YT, Cornblath M, Sidbury JB. Cornstarch therapy in type 1 glycogen-storage disease. N Engl J Med 1984;310:1721-1725.

3. Kaufman FR, Devgan S. Use of uncooked cornstarch to avert nocturnal hypoglycemia in children and adolescents with type 1 diabetes. J Diabetes Compl 1996;10:84-87.

4. Kaufman FR, Halvorson M, Kaufman ND. A randomized, blinded trial of uncooked cornstarch to diminish nocturnal hypoglycemia at diabetes camp. Diabetes Research and Clinical Practice 1995; 30:205-209.

5. Kaufman FR, Halvorson M, Kaufman ND. Evaluation of a snack bar containing uncooked cornstarch in subjects with diabetes. Diabetes Research and Clinical Practice in press.

HYPOALLERGENIC FORMULATIONS AND MEDICAL FOODS, THE NEOCATE PRODUCT RANGE

Mark A. De Fries,
Chief Executive Officer
SHS North America
Rockville
Maryland

SHS North America ("SHS"), located in Rockville, Maryland is a twelve (12) year old subsidiary of SHS International based in Liverpool, England. SHS International and its subsidiaries are wholly owned by Nutricia B.V. of Zoetermeer, The Netherlands. Mark De Fries, the Chief Executive Officer and also a board member has been with SHS since 1985. As the head of North American operation since 1985, Mr. De Fries faced some difficult and unique challenges and has championed the technology and clinical trials to commercialize nutritional products in Medical Food arena. Among the topics to be discuss in this case study are the following:

Medical Foods - Outline of Presentation

- History and Overview of the Company
- Medical Foods Positioning
- Medical Foods Definition and Regulations
- Product line / Hypoallergenic Formulations
- Neocate One + Market Niche
- Features and Comparisons
- Clinical Trials
- Trials to Commercialization
- Keys to Success
- Summary of Results of Neocate Product Range

History and Overview of the Company

The history of SHS commences in 1879 with the establishment of Powell and Schoelfield Ltd., a Liverpool based manufacturer of brewing additives, by the banks of the Mersey

River and in close proximity to Albert Dock, the main shipping port of the Northwest section of England.

In the early 1960's, SHS Ltd. was established as a manufacturer of defined dietary treatments used in the clinical intervention of rare amino acid metabolic disorders. While SHS Ltd. served many disease specific markets, a handful of specialized nutritional products diseases made up a greater percentage of their sales and profits.

In 1985 SHS Ltd. embarked on their globalization strategy with the incorporation of SHS Inc. Starting with $5000 of inventory and the prospects of the United States Inborn Error market, the corporation built the market for the products to approximately $1MM in sales in two years.

The U.K. Parent Corporation, seeing the potential of the rapid growth in sales, accepted the approaches by Ross Laboratories (Abbott International), Infant Formula Division, and signed an exclusive 5-year license/distribution agreement to sell SHS name branded products. Ross used these specialized products as a marketing tool, to promote their infant formula (IF) product. Ross, playing in the fiercely competitive IF market, believed that the SHS product line would enhance the scientific image of the Ross product.

As of December 31, 1992, Ross elected not to renew the license/distribution agreement with SHS Ltd. and as a result SHS Inc. once again focused its attention on this core business. Ross is now a direct competitor of SHS Inc., since they have developed a competing product line.

As a result of the aforementioned distribution transfer, SHS' 1994-5 product line consisted of approximately two dozen FDA approved products classified as medical foods used in the treatment of inherited metabolic diseases. Originally conceived of in the 1960s but having gone through constant revisions, this product line remains the core business area of SHS through the 1990s.

SHS' sole dependence on the inherited metabolic disease product line posed strategic and competitive marketing liabilities due to technological improvements, genetic engineering, and improved prenatal diagnostic techniques. The reliance on a single market was a threat to SHS, restricting company growth and expansion potential. Additionally, large multi-national conglomerates and competitors such as Mead Johnson and Ross Laboratories (makers of Similac, Isomil, Pregestimil and Alimentum) have resources far in excess to compete in new markets and new product development. In short, SHS was faced with the eventuality that our existing product line would face a declining market. It was the strategic direction of the organization in 1992 to enter an unrelated market to further strengthen the corporation. SHS was challenged to develop a new strategic market by 1996 while retaining and maturing the core business area.

The potential of a special hypoallergenic infant formula was attractive in that the market in the United States represents between $82-$100 million dollars. This financial growth could be achieved while having an overall impact on infant nutritional well being and often results in saving infant life.

History and Overview of the Company

- **1879 Formed Powell & Scholefield**
  - Brewing Additives Business
- **1960 Formed Scientific Hospital Supplies**
  - Metabolic Formulations for Inborn Errors of Metabolism
- **1985 Incorporated SHS North America**
  - Metabolic Formulations for Inborn Errors of Metabolism
- **1990 - 1991 Set out Plans for Diversification in Hypoallergenic Market**
- **1994 - 1995 Commercialization of Hypoallergenic Products**

Figure 1.

A summary of the chronology of the history of the corporation and major areas of business opportunities is presented in Figure 1.

Medical Foods Positioning

SHS North America is positioned within clinical nutrition and that falls somewhere between the food industry and the drug industry. Medical Foods are positioned somewhere in this area (See Figure 2) although the actual location is a matter of dispute and concern.

Medical Foods Definition and Regulations

Although communicated throughout this seminar, I believe the basic definition and regulations surrounding this class of product require reiteration. A medical foods is formulated to be consumed or administered enterally under the supervision of a physician and is intended for the specific dietary management of a disease or condition for which distinctive nutritional requirements, based on recognized scientific principals, are established by medical evaluation, more specifically:

- It is specifically formulated and processed for the partial or exclusive feeding of a patient
- It is intended for the dietary management of a patient who, because of therapeutic or chronic medical needs, has limited or impaired capacity to ingest, digest, absorb, or metabolize ordinary foodstuffs or certain nutrients, or who has special medically determined nutrient requirement, the dietary management of which cannot be achieved by the modification of normal diet alone;
- It provide nutritional support specifically modified for the management of the unique nutrient needs that result from the specific disease or condition, as determined by medical evaluation:

Medical Foods Positioning

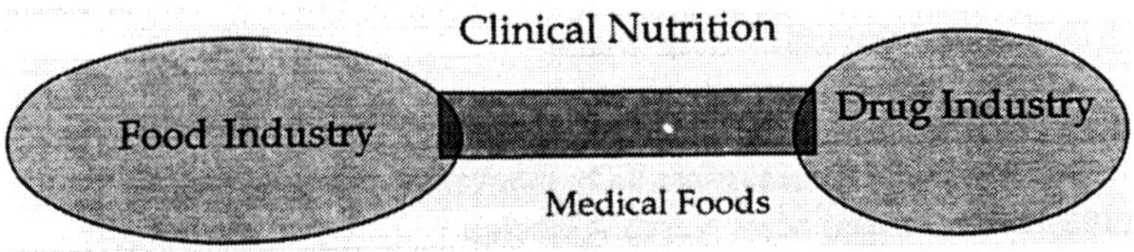

Figure 2.

- It is intended to be used under medical supervision. It is intended only for a patient receiving active and ongoing medical supervision wherein the patient requires medical care on a recurring basis for, among other things, instructions on the use of the medical food.

As far as the regulatory issues that are involved with theses product, the FDA has not published anything that defines medical foods other than what has appeared in the Federal Register. The Agency is considering regulations of medical foods as defined by the Orphan Drug Act.

The concept of "medical foods" was first given legal status as a separate regulatory entity when it was defined in the Orphan Drug Amendments to the Code of Regulations of 1988 of the Federal Food, Drug and Cosmetic Act. President Bush incorporated it into the Nutrition Labeling and Education Act of 1990.

For many years the FDA has been publishing the following statement in the Federal Register, but medical food regulations remain unpublished:

"The Food and Drug Administration is considering development of regulations for medical foods, as defined by the Orphan Drug Act Amendments of 1988 (21 USC 360ee (b) (3)) to assure, among other things, the safety and effectiveness of these product, proper labeling of the nutrient content and purposed uses, including adequate and appropriate directions for use, quality control and good manufacturing practices."

Product line / Hypoallergenic Formulations

The evaluation of reactions and ultimate treatment after the ingestion of foods is one of the more challenging and controversial topics in allergy and gastroentrology. The clinical management of food allergy is predicated on the identification and removal of the offending food product and the treatment of the adverse reactions. Food allergy has been variously estimated from 0.3% to 7.5% in children and the incidence decreases with age (Gerrard, J.W. et al, Acta Paediatr Scand, 1973; 1-21).

Product line / Hypoallergenic Formulations

Exempt Infant Formula - Neocate

- Medical Food - over the age of 1 year
  - Neocate One + Liquid
  - Neocate One + Powdered
- Medical Food - over the age of 5 and Adult formulation
  - EO 28 Extra

Figure 3.

Neocate One Plus, as an hypoallergenic, elemental juvenile formula, is ideally suited to this market as a ready-to-feed (RTF)Tetra-Pak product, with an acceptable taste.

Currently, there are competitors that control substantial market share of the entire infant hypoallergenic business. However, there is reason to believe that no major pharmaceutical, infant formula manufacturer, or consumer food manufacturer will be able to effectively capture the current Neocate market (See Figure 3.), due to its relatively technical nature. During the early stages of developing this market, SHS must carefully position itself as a disease specific formula manufacturer and not a generic producer.

Neocate One + Market Niche

Product development of novel niche products depends on creativity. Generic formula producers responded to their competitors in introduction of new products and "unique" concepts. SHS' market success depends upon inventions by internal or collaborative R & D and \ or "market support" by small groups of academic collaborators \ scientists working in an essentially entrepreneurial mode; this is one of our advantages over the large multi-national corporations.

Marketing costs are relatively high for niche marketing organizations. A niche market organization routinely spends 20-30% or more of their sales on sales and marketing activities, this is at least in part due to the immaturity of distribution channels. Brand name, customer service, market leadership, size and image are very important in this market. Generally, niche market leaders grow more powerful as a function of time: the distribution channels and end users favor them over larger competitors simply because of market identification and support to a subsection of a larger market.

Features and Comparisons

The unique ready-to-feed Amino Acid formulation of Neocate One +, differentiates the product from other elemental or semi-elemental formulas currently on the market. The superior palatability issue of Neocate One +, further separates SHS' product from the competitors. Additionally, Neocate One + by design, clinical results, and placement within a defined market; as an age and disease specific formulation, are among the unique attributes of this product.

Clinical Trials

SHS Inc. has developed an unique corporate / academic clinical relationship with Johns Hopkins Medical Center, Department of Pediatrics - Division of Gastroentrology and Nutrition to evaluate Neocate One + within this center of excellence. The clinical study is designed to study the possibility that children may have unsuspected allergies to commonly ingested food proteins. These allergies may be responsible for common upper stomach symptoms such as vomiting, loss of appetite, nausea, diarrhea, weight loss, and food refusal behavior. The study will also investigate the relationship between the presence of eosinophils found on mucosal biopsies to these aforementioned symptoms. The Divisions of GI / Nutrition and Allergy and Immunology are collaborating in this study.

The results of this study will be key to the success of the technical marketing efforts required to promote this product to the medical community worldwide. Since the original publication of Neocate (Sampson, H.A. et al *Journal Of Pediatrics*, September 1992,463-464) SHS Inc has seen a dramatic increase in the demand for Neocate. The process of world class clinical trials being conducted and journal articles published on SHS products are paramount to the successful marketing of technologically superior clinical nutritional products worldwide.

The results of the clinical trial are reported by Dr. Kelly *et al.* entitled, Eosinophilic esophagitis attributed to gastroesopageal relux: improvement with an amino acid-based formulas. (**Gastroenterology** 1995; 109:1503-12).

Trials to Commercialization

SHS North America will be focusing on the Immunological / Allergist and Gastroenterologists market for Neocate One +. The initial marketing will be in the form of poster presentations, seminars, workshops, and initial professional personal communications.

The initial strategy for the launching of Neocate One +, will be "scientific breakthrough" journal reports indicating the benefit of a specific elemental diet in the treatment of defined food allergies. Close contact with our customer base will determine potentially interested physicians (our innovators or 20% of the population) to determine target centers. Figure 4 attempts to detail some of the marketing activities necessary to bring the Neocate range of products to commercialization. SHS North America will be focusing on a new business area and efforts to develop this market should be functionally separate from our current core business area, yet administratively supported from SHS Inc.

Trials to Commercialization

- "Message" to Target Audience
- Production
- Physical Form
- Labeling
- Claims
- Literature
- Sales force preparation
- Production forecast - Initial Inventory Levels
- Distribution patterns

Figure 4.

Keys to Success

SHS Inc. believes that the keys to success in this business are:

- Clinically proven at world recognized institution and published results in peer review journal of 100% hypoallergenic RTF formula specifically designed for Pediatric use in at risk individuals
- Distribution: by dealing with the distribution channels in a non-traditional manner
- Product Quality and Appearance: To appeal to the adolescent both in formulation and packaging design.
- Management: Products delivered on time, cost controlled, and marketing budgets managed. There is temptation to fix on growth at the expense of profits.

Summary of Results of Neocate Product Range

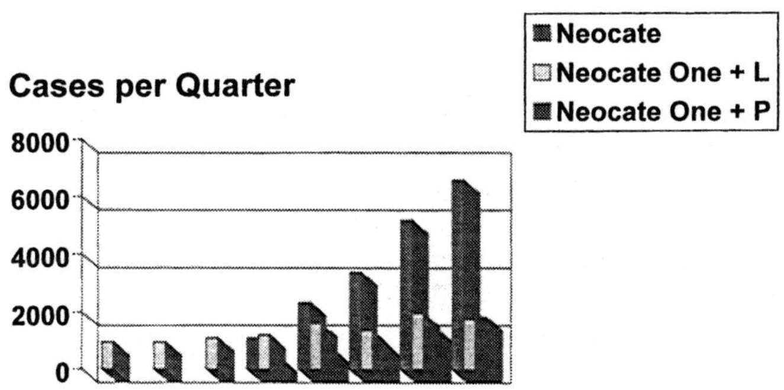

APPENDIX I Advance Notice of Proposed Rulemaking

DEPARTMENT OF HEALTH AND HUMAN SERVICES

Food and Drug Administration

21 CFR Ch. I.

[Docket No. 96N-0364]

RIN 0905-AD91

Regulation of Medical Foods

AGENCY: Food and Drug Administration, HHS.

ACTION: Advance notice of proposed rulemaking.

SUMMARY: The Food and Drug Administration (FDA) is soliciting comments to initiate a reevaluation of its approach to the regulation of the broad group of heterogeneous products that are marketed as medical foods. FDA's goal is to arrive at a regulatory regime that will ensure that: These products are safe for their intended uses, especially because they are likely to be the sole or a major source of nutrients for sick and otherwise vulnerable people; claims for these products are truthful, not misleading, and supported by sound science; and the labeling of these products is adequate to inform consumers about how to use them in a safe and appropriate manner. The agency believes that there is a need to reevaluate its policy for regulating medical foods because of a number of developments, including enactment of a statutory definition of "medical food," the rapid increase in the variety and number of products that are marketed as medical foods, safety problems associated with the manufacture and quality control of these products, and the potential for fraud as claims that are not supported by sound science proliferate for these products.

DATES: Written comments by February 27, 1997.

ADDRESSES: Submit written comments to the Dockets Management Branch (HFA-305), Food and Drug Administration, 12420 Parklawn Dr., rm. 1-23, Rockville, MD 20857. Submit written requests for single copies of FDA's Compliance Program for Medical Foods (Compliance Program No. 7321.002) to the Freedom of Information Office (HFI-35), Food and Drug Administration, 5600 Fishers Lane, Rockville, MD 20857. Send two self-addressed adhesive labels to assist that office in processing your requests.

FOR FURTHER INFORMATION CONTACT:
Robert J. Moore, Center for Food Safety and Applied Nutrition (HFS-456), Food and Drug Administration, 200 C St. SW., Washington, DC 20204, 202-205-4605.

SUPPLEMENTARY INFORMATION

I. Background

One of the first medical foods to be developed was the infant formula Lofenalac®, a product that was designed for use in the dietary management of a rare genetic condition known as phenylketonuria (PKU). This product contains only a very limited amount of the essential amino acid phenylalanine because the individuals with this condition have an impaired ability to metabolize this amino acid. If infants with PKU consume foods that contain phenylalanine, harmful end products of phenylalanine metabolism accumulate in the body and can cause severe, irreversible mental retardation. Dietary management to carefully limit phenylalanine intake (for example, by using a formula that provides only a limited, minimal amount of this essential amino acid) can result in normal growth and development and avoid mental retardation.

Before 1972, FDA regulated products like the infant formula Lofenalac® as drugs under section 201(g)(1)(B) of the Federal Food, Drug. and Cosmetic Act (the act) (21 U.S.C. 321(g)(1)(B)) because of their role in mitigating serious adverse effects of the underlying diseases. In 1972, FDA reassessed its position. At that time, such products were very limited in number and were being produced by a small number of reputable manufacturers with high standards of quality control. Additionally, the nutritional formulation requirements for this type of product were straightforward and well established by the medical community. FDA believed that the usefulness of these products in patient populations was widely accepted by health care professionals, and that close physician supervision ensured safe use in the patient population. The agency was interested in fostering innovation In the development of these products, most of which had been developed for the dietary management of diseases and conditions that are not widespread, to ensure that such products would be available at reasonable cost. For all these reasons, the agency concluded that a revision of its regulatory approach to these products was appropriate. At the same time, the agency recognized that use of these products for feeding healthy individuals could be hazardous. For example, an infant formula that was purposely formulated to be suitable for an infant with PKU would be nutritionally inadequate for a normal infant. Thus, the agency saw that it was important to differentiate these products from foods for general use. As a result, in 1972, FDA stated that the PKU product described above would no longer be regulated as a drug but rather as a "food for special dietary use"[1] (37 FR 18229 at 18230, September 8, 1972). In addition, the agency began to follow a policy of regulating similar types of products as foods for special dietary use.

---

[1]Although there was no statutory definition of a food for special dietary use in 1972, the term "special dietary uses," as applied to food for humans, had been defined by regulation since 1941. In the Federal Register of November 22, 1941 (6 FR 59211, FDA promulgated a regulation stating that the term "special dietary uses". as applied to food for man, means particular (as distinguished from
(continued)

Since 1972, the legislative and regulatory history of medical foods has reflected the agency's efforts to develop a regulatory framework to ensure the safety and nutritional adequacy of foods that are designed to meet distinctive nutritional requirements resulting from diseases or health conditions. Medical foods are used under the supervision of a physician when such distinctive nutritional requirements cannot be met with a conventional diet. These characteristics have led the agency to exempt medical foods from many of the requirements that apply to conventional foods.

When FDA made nutrition labeling mandatory for certain foods in 1973, the agency exempted certain types of foods for special dietary use from this requirement. In the preamble to the 1973 final rule on nutrition labeling (38 FR 2124 at 2126, January 19, 1973), FDA noted that nutrition labeling developed for foods intended for consumption by the general population was not well suited for some food products, including two types of foods for special dietary use: (1) Any food represented for use as the sole item of the diet; and (2) foods represented for use solely under medical supervision in the dietary management of specific diseases and disorders. Therefore, this final rule provided that these two types of foods for special dietary use would be exempt from the general requirements for nutrition labeling and were to be labeled in compliance with regulations that the agency intended to include in 21 CFR part 125 (later designated as 21 CFR part 105).

The Orphan Drug Amendments of 1988 enacted, for the first time, a statutory definition of "medical food":

> The term "medical food" means a food which is formulated to be consumed or administered enterally under the supervision of a physician and which is intended for the specific dietary management of a disease or condition for which distinctive nutritional requirements, based on recognized scientific principles, are established by medical evaluation.

(21 U.S.C. 360ee(b)(3))

Although Congress provided a statutory definition for medical foods, the legislative history of the Orphan Drug Amendments does not discuss the definition and, therefore, does not provide any further information regarding the types of products that the definition was intended to cover.

---

general) uses of food, and that it means. among other things, "uses for supplying particular dietary needs which exist by reason of a physical, physiological, pathological or other condition, including but not limited to the conditions of disease, convalescence, pregnancy. lactation, allergic hypersensitivity to food, underweight. and overweight." This part of the regulation remains unchanged is current §105.3(a)(l)(21 CFR 105. 3(a)(1)).

The statutory definition of "special dietary use" in section 411(c)(3) of the act (21 U.S.C. 350(c)(3)) was added in 1976 (Pub. L. 94-278). It defines this term as a particular use for which a food purports or is represented to be used, including but not limited to the following:

(A) Supplying a special dietary need that exists by reason of a physical, physiological, pathological, or other condition, including but not limited to the condition of disease, convalescence. pregnancy, lactation, infancy, allergic hypersensitivity to food, underweight, overweight, or the need to control intake of sodium.

(B) Supplying a vitamin, mineral, or other ingredient for use by man to supplement his diet by increasing the total dietary intake.

(C)Supplying a special dietary need by reason of being a food for use as the sole item of the diet.

In the Nutrition Labeling and Education Act of 1990 (the 1990 amendments), Congress incorporated the definition of medical foods contained in the Orphan Drug Amendments of 1988 into section 403(q)(5)(A)(iv) of the act (21 U.S.C. 343(q)(5)(A)(iv)) and exempted medical foods from the nutrition labeling, health claim, and nutrient content claim requirements applicable to most other foods. In the Federal Register of November 27, 1991 (56 FR 60366 at 60377), FDA published a proposal to implement the mandatory nutrition labeling provisions of the 1990 amendments. The proposal discussed the statutory exemption for medical foods and advised that the agency considered the statutory definition of medical foods to "narrowly constrain the types of products that can be considered to fall within this exemption." In the Federal Register of January 6, 1993, FDA published several final rules implementing the 1990 amendments. The final rule on mandatory nutrition labeling (58 FR 2079 at 2151, January 6, 1993) exempted medical foods from the nutrition labeling requirements and incorporated the statutory definition of a medical food into the agency's regulations at §101.9(j)(8) (21 CFR 101.9(j)(8). In this regulation, FDA enumerated criteria that were intended to clarify the characteristics of medical foods. The regulation provides that a food may claim the exemption from nutrition labeling requirements only if it meets the following criteria in§101.9(j)(8):

(I) It is a specially formulated and processed product (as opposed to a naturally occurring foodstuff used in its natural state) for the partial or exclusive feeding of a patient by means of oral intake orenteral feeding by tube;

(ii) It is intended for the dietary management of a patient who, because of therapeutic or chronic medical needs, has limited or impaired capacity to ingest, digest, absorb, or metabolize ordinary foodstuffs or certain nutrients, or who has other special medically determined nutrient requirements, the dietary management of which cannot be achieved by the modification of the normal diet alone;

(iii) It provides nutritional support specifically modified for the management of the unique[2] nutrient needs that result from the specific disease or condition, as determined by medical evaluation;

(iv) It is intended to be used under medical supervision; and

(v) It is intended only for a patient receiving active and ongoing medical supervision wherein the patient requires medical care on a recurring basis for, among other things, instructions on the use of the medical food.

(58 FR 2079 at 2185)

In the preamble to the final rule on mandatory nutrition labeling, FDA noted that it had received a number of comments asking for further clarification of the types of products that the agency considers to be medical foods. The agency

---

[2]The agency notes that experience has shown that the word that it should have used here is "distinctive" rather than "unique." Thus, in any rulemaking that results from the advance notice of proposed rulemaking, the agency will likely propose to amend§101.9(j)(8) accordingly.

acknowledged that such clarification would be helpful and announced that it intended to address the issue in the future (58 FR 2079 at 2151). In the same document, the agency also noted the need for labeling regulations for medical foods and reiterated its intention to propose such regulations.

In 1990, the Life Sciences Research Office of the Federation of American Societies for Experimental Biology (LSRO/FASEB) published "Guidelines for the Scientific Review of Enteral Food Products for Special Medical Purposes" (Ref. 1). This report defined medical foods as products that are distinct from foods for special dietary use in that they "demonstrate greater suitability for nutritional management of a specific disease than standard enteral formulas" and are intended for patients with "special medically determined nutrient requirements, the dietary management of whom cannot be achieved by the modification of the normal diet alone, by other foods for special dietary uses, or by a combination thereof." The report proposed criteria that would establish a strict standard that a food would have to meet to be considered a medical food. LSRO /FASEB's proposed definition of a medical food did not include all foods that might be useful for persons with a disease or medical condition.

II. Reasons for Re-Evaluating Regulation of Medical Foods

A. *Introduction*

The agency is re-evaluating its policy for regulating medical foods in light of several developments, including the enactment of a statutory definition of "medical food," the impact of the 1990 amendments, the rapid increase in the variety and number of products that are marketed as medical foods and in the uses for which these products are marketed, safety problems associated with the manufacture and quality control of these products, and the resulting potential for injury to consumers and fraud as claims that are not supported by sound science proliferate for these products.

B. *The Definition of "Medical Food" and the Impact of the 1990 Amendments: the Medical Foods Paradox*

The statutory definitions of "medical food" (21 U.S.C. 360ee(b)(3)) and food for special dietary use (see section 411 (c) (3) of the act), and the differing treatment of these two categories of products under the 1990 amendments to the act (i.e., medical foods are exempted under section 403(q)(5)(A)(iv) and special treatment of foods for special dietary use), establish that Congress intended and medical foods and foods for special dietary use be viewed and regulated as separator and distinct categories of products. Foods for special dietary use are subject to the same nutrition labeling requirements and nutrient content claims established for most other foods by the 1990 amendments. Thus, foods for special dietary use, like ordinary foods, must be labeled with certain nutrition information in a prescribed format to ensure that such information is presented in an informative and understandable fashion. Moreover, any nutrient content claims or health claims on the label or in the labeling of a food for special dietary use must have been authorized by FDA to ensure that the claim is scientifically valid and is presented in such a way that it is truthful and not misleading.

In contrast, under the 1990 amendments, medical foods are specifically exempted from the requirements for nutrition labeling, nutrient content claims, and health claims. Thus, a medical food that is intended for the specific dietary management of a disease or condition for which distinctive nutritional requirements have been established may be sold without any nutrition information on its label or labeling, and it may bear claims that have not been evaluated under the 1990 amendments to ensure that they are scientifically valid. Moreover, there is no assurance that the formulation of a medical food has been evaluated prior to sale to ensure that it is suitable for the intended patient population. The exemption from the requirements of the 1990 amendments, therefore, creates a troubling paradox: Medical foods intended for use by sick people are subject to much less scrutiny than virtually all other foods, which are intended for the healthy general population. This lack of scrutiny creates a situation that could have adverse public health consequences if theseproducts bear claims that are not scientifically valid; or if their labeling does not disclose nutrition or other information that is necessary for the safe and effective use of the food.

C. *Universe of Products*

The number and variety of products marketed as medical foods, the number and types of claims made for such products, the types of ingredients included in these products, and the number of manufacturers of these products have increased significantly since the mid-1970's. In 1974, a limited survey of pharmaceutical and food manufacturers revealed that fewer than three dozen products were being sold as medical foods (Ref. 2). As of 1989, however, well over 200 products were being sold as medical foods (Ref. 3). Table I lists several types of products being marketed as medical foods with examples of claims being made by vendors of these products.

However, many products marketed as medical foods may not qualify as such under the statutory definition of medical foods. Many of these products, for example, complete liquid nutrition products, are not formulated or promoted for the dietary management of a particular disease or condition but rather are formulated and marketed for use by the general population as supplements to a normal diet or as meal replacements.

Enteral nutrition is nutrition provided through the gastrointestinal tract, taken by mouth or provided through a tube or catheter that delivers nutrients beyond the oral cavity (i.e., directly to the stomach or small intestine). This document uses the term "enteral nutrition products" to refer to products that have been marketed as medical foods, "statutory medical foods" to refer to enteral nutrition products that meet the statutory definition of a medical food in section 5(b)(3) of the Orphan Drug Amendments (21 U.S.C. 360ee(b)(3)); and "nonstatutory enteral nutrition products" to refer to enteral nutrition products that have been marketed as medical foods but that do not meet the statutory definition of a medical food.

Enteral nutrition products labeled and marketed as medical foods are generally liquid or powdered products formulated to meet specific needs. They include nutritionally complete formulations, nutritionally incomplete formulations (such as modular products that contain only one nutrient or a small number of nutrients and that are intended for use with other formulations), formulations for metabolic disorders (including inborn errors of metabolism) in patients over 12 months of age, and oral rehydration products. While many such products are intended to provide a complete source of nutrition and are consumed orally or

TABLE 1.—EXAMPLES OF CURRENTLY AVAILABLE TYPES OF ENTERAL NUTRITION PRODUCTS FOR USE IN VARIOUS DISEASE STATES AND FOR PATIENTS WITH INBORN ERRORS OF METABOLISM[1]

Disease state	Patient population	Product characteristics	Examples of product claims
Kidney (renal) disease (e.g., chronic or acute kidney failure).	Hospitalized patients (including critical care patients) and home care patients.	Type and quality of protein.	"* * * complete balanced nutrition for renal patients * * * a moderate-protein, low-electrolyte, low-fluid, high-calorie formula * * * designed to provide balanced-nutrition for dialyzed patients with chronic or acute renal failure * * *" "Under careful dietary management * * * can maintain uremic patients in good nutritional status, promote anabolism and lower and stabilize blood urea nitrogen levels * * *"
Liver disease (e.g., coma or encephalopathy associated with hepatitis or cirrhosis).	Hospitalized patients (including critical care patients) and home care patients.	Type and quality of protein.	"Provides adequate protein without inducing or exacerbating hepatic encephalopathy" An aggressive nutritional regimen * * * may be useful in the nutritional management of alcoholic liver-disease patients in reversing malnutrition, liver dysfunction, and encephalopathy."
Hypermetabolic states (e.g., severe burns, trauma or infection).	Hospitalized patients (including critical care patients).	Type and quality of protein; added amino acids; elevated levels of specific vitamins and/or minerals.	"A nutritionally complete formula that provides a concentrated source of calories for patients with restricted fluid allowance or increased energy needs * * * useful in the dietary management of volume-restricted patients, oncology patients, hypermetabolic conditions, trauma, sepsis, and post major surgery." "Specialized elemental nutrition with glutamine for metabolically stressed patients with impaired GI function * * * stimulates intestinal epithelial cell proliferation in injured rats * * * diminished mucosal atrophy associated with injury by stimulating intestinal cell replacement."
Lung disease (e.g., chronic obstructive pulmonary disease, acute respiratory distress syndrome, cystic fibrosis).	Hospitalized patients (including critical care patients) and home care patients.	High fat, low carbohydrate content.	"A nutritionally complete, ready-to-use formula * * * uniquely formulated to provide a diet high in nitrogen and restricted in carbohydrates to aid in the control of metabolic alterations in * * * various stress states including respiratory insufficiency * * * CO_2 production is minimized while providing appropriate nutrient levels." "Proven effective in the dietary management of patients with respiratory disease * * * reduced CO_2 production in chronic obstructive pulmonary disease and cystic fibrosis patients."

(continued)

TABLE 1.—EXAMPLES OF CURRENTLY AVAILABLE TYPES OF ENTERAL NUTRITION PRODUCTS FOR USE IN VARIOUS DISEASE STATES AND FOR PATIENTS WITH INBORN ERRORS OF METABOLISM [1]—Continued

Disease state	Patient population	Product characteristics	Examples of product claims
Compromised immune function. Human immunodeficiency virus (HIV) infection, acquired immune deficiency syndrome (AIDS).	Hospitalized patients (including critical care patients) and home care patients.	Enriched with specific amino acids; fortified with increased levels of vitamins.	"Specialized complete nutrition to provide effective nutritional management for people with HIV infection or AIDS * * * to support immune function." "Increases CD_4/CD_8 ratio, one aspect of immune system * * * CD_4/CD_8 increased by day 5, indicating an improved T-helper cell function." "7 days of use helped support return of immune function to preoperative levels; 22 percent reduction in mean length of hospital stay; 70 percent reduction in infections and wound complications."
Diabetes mellitus	Hospitalized patients (including critical care patients) and home care patients.	Type and quantity of carbohydrate; high fiber.	"High fiber, low carbohydrate * * * for patients with abnormal glucose tolerance * * * to enhance blood glucose control * * * in persons with type I or type II diabetes mellitus and stress-induced hyperglycemia."
Malabsorption, as found in: Inflammatory bowel disease (ulcerative colitis, Crohn's disease); radiation enteritis; short bowel syndrome.	Hospitalized patients (including critical care patients) and home care patients.	Pre-digested macronutrients; altered type or quantity of fat.	"A nutritionally complete enteral nutritional with * * * 85 percent of fat derived from (medium chain triglyceride) (MCT) oil—a lipid clinically proven to result in less severity and incidence of diarrhea and abdominal discomfort in individuals with fat malabsorption * * * resulting from conditions such as HIV infection, inflammatory bowel disease, cystic fibrosis, or short bowel syndrome." "Comparision of a semi-elemental diet with Prednisolone in the primary treatment of active ileal Crohn's disease * * * this new flavored semi-elemental diet * * * may be as effective as steroids in inducing remission in ideal Crohn's disease."
Oral rehydration solutions	Hospitalized patients (including critical care patients) and home care patients.	Solutions of water, electrolytes and a carbohydrate source.	"To quickly restore fluids and minerals lost in diarrhea and vomiting in infants and children * * * for maintenance of water and electrolytes following corrective parenteral therapy for severe diarrhea." "Enteral rehydration solution * * * to prevent dehydration and to correct mild to moderate dehydration associated with fluid and electrolyte loss." "Pediatric electrolyte oral maintenance solution * * * to restore body water and minerals lost in children's diarrhea and vomiting * * * prevents dehydration."

Phenylketonuria (PKU)	Patients with phenylketonuria.	Restrict dietary phenylalanine.	"A phenylalanine-free food to aid in the nutritional management of hyperphenylalaninemia including PKU." "Phenylalanine-free to allow greater intake of complete protein." "Phenylalanine-free for pregnant women, women in the childbearing years and individuals over 8 years of age."
Maple syrup urine disease	Patients with maple syrup urine disease.	Restrict dietary branched-chain amino acids (isoleucine, leucine and valine).	"To be used only for the dietary management of infants and children with maple syrup urine disease or other disorders of branched-chain amino acid metabolism under the direct and continuing supervision of a physician." "A branched-chain amino acid-free medical food * * * for nutrition support of children and adults with branch-chain ketoaciduria (maple syrup urine disease)." "Isoleucine-, leucine- and valine-free for individuals over 8 years of age and women in the childbearing years."
Hereditary tyrosinemia: Type I Type II.	Patients with hereditary tyrosinemia.	For Type I: Restrict dietary tyrosine, phenylalanine and methionine;. For Type II: Restrict dietary tyrosine and phenylalanine.	"A phenylalanine-, tyrosine- and methionine-free medical food * * * for nutrition support of infants and toddlers with tyrosinemia type I." "A special formula powder for use in the dietary management of hereditary tyrosinemia II * * * a phenylalanine- and tyrosine-free medical food for nutrition support of children and adults with tyrosinemia type II." "A special formula powder for use in the dietary management of hereditary tyrosinemia II * * * very low in tyrosine and phenylalanine * * * "
Homocystinuria	Patients with homocystinuria.	Restrict dietary methionine.	"A special diet powder without added methionine for dietary management of individuals with homocystinuria." "A methionine-free medical food * * * for nutritional support of children and adults with vitamin B_6-nonresponsive homocystinuria or hypermethioninemia,"

(continued)

TABLE 1.—EXAMPLES OF CURRENTLY AVAILABLE TYPES OF ENTERAL NUTRITION PRODUCTS FOR USE IN VARIOUS DISEASE STATES AND FOR PATIENTS WITH INBORN ERRORS OF METABOLISM[1]—Continued

Disease state	Patient population	Product characteristics	Examples of product claims
			"Methionine-free for individuals over 8 years of age and women in the childbearing years."
Urea cycle disorders (e.g., argininemia, ornithine transcarbamylase deficiency, methylmalonic aciduria).	Patients with urea cycle disorders.	Restrict dietary protein as tolerated without causing hyperammonemia.	"A non-essential amino acid-free medical food * * * for nutrition support of children and adults with a defect in a urea cycle enzyme * * *"

[1] This is a summary description of products available for dietary management of the listed diseases and inborn errors of metabolism. Some of these diseases and conditions have many variations, each requiring distinctive dietary restrictions or supplements to the diet. A number of products are available for several of the listed diseases and conditions, and the actual composition of these products may vary slightly from the product characteristics given in this summary.

administered by feeding tube for this use, the labeling of such products frequently bears claims related to an intended use of the product in the management of a disease or condition, e.g., in alleviating specific symptoms and clinical manifestations of a particular disease.

D. Safety Problems

As discussed above, there has been a dramatic increase over the past 20 years in the number and types of products that purport to be medical foods. The number of manufacturers producing these products has also increased. As the number of manufacturers has grown, the level of industry experience in the current good manufacturing practice -(CGMP) and quality control procedures necessary to produce products that contain nutrients within a narrow range of declared label values has become quite variable. Medical foods are complex formulated products, generally requiring sophisticated and exacting technology comparable to that used in the manufacture of infant formulas and drugs. Moreover, the populations that consume these products, often as the sole or a major source of nutrition, are extremely vulnerable, e.g., pediatric patients in periods of growth and development, the elderly, patients who have serious illnesses, and patients in intensive care units. Although excessive or, conversely, insufficient amounts of particular nutrients may not be a health hazard when consumed by healthy persons, serious adverse consequences (even death) may result when these vulnerable populations consume these products for long, or even short, periods of time.

Significantly, in recent years, FDA has become aware of some serious problems with foods that purport to be medical foods. In 1986, four infants died as a result of being fed an oral rehydration solution that contained lethal concentrations of potassium. FDA identified the oral rehydration solution as the cause of these deaths (Ref. 4), inspected the site where the product was manufactured, and analyzed the product's nutrient content. FDA determined that elevated amounts of potassium occurred in the product because CGMP had not been followed. Notably, weighing scales were used improperly, and persons responsible for the formulation of product lacked adequate training.

Results of a compliance program that FDA initiated for medical foods in 1988, andfollowup on adverse reactions reported to the agency, have identified examples of deviations from CGMP that have caused the actual nutrient content of the product to deviate significantly from the declared label value. Some deviations have been significant enough to create acute, life-threatening health hazards and have led to product recalls. For example, in 1989, problems with a nutritionally complete product containing excessive amounts of potassium and sodium were brought to FDA's attention as a result of a complaint from the Veterans Administration Medical Center in Nashville, TN. Administration of this product to a patient resulted in hyperkalemia, or elevated blood potassium levels, which can have life threatening consequences, including fatal cardiac arrhythmias. This patient required intensive medical treatment to reduce blood potassium levels and to prevent the serious side effects of hyperkalemia. FDA inspection of the facility that had manufactured this product revealed serious flaws in CGMP. These flaws resulted in extreme variability in product composition between lots or individual packets of product, which became evident when the product was analyzed by FDA for nutrient composition. This product was recalled (Ref. 5).

In 1993, in response to a complaint to FDA from a medical center in Seattle, WA, FDA analysis of a complete nutritional product being administered enterally to patients in an intensive care unit revealed that the product contained levels of potassium that were approximately twice the amount declared on the label, The agency concluded that this product represented an acute, potentially life-threatening hazard to persons with impaired kidney function, particularly those who were not being closely monitored for serum potassium levels. As a result, a number of products were recalled (Ref. 6).

FDA is also aware of problems involving potential microbiological contamination of products that purport to be medical foods. For example, in 1993, a modular product containing protein and a modular product containing carbohydrate were recalled because they had been manufactured under conditions in which they may have become contaminated with *Salmonella* (Ref. 7).

E. Claims and the Potential for Economic Fraud

FDA has not, to date, undertaken a comprehensive review of the claims being made for products that purport to be medical foods but rather has evaluated claims for a small number of these products on a case-by-case basis, applying the following general principles:

1. A product marketed for use as a medical food in the dietary management of a disease or condition should have characteristics that are based on scientifically validated distinctive nutritional requirements of the disease or condition.
2. There should be a scientific basis for the formulation of the product and the claims made for the product.
3. There should be sound, scientifically defensible evidence that the product does what it claims to do.

The agency is concerned that some of the claims made for products that purport to be medical foods are not based on sound science, and that consumers that use products that bear such claims, and health professionals that recommend the use of such products, are being misled regarding the value of these products. In addition to the health risks created by unsafe or ineffective medical foods, consumers and third-party payers, such as insurance companies and government health care agencies, suffer significant economic losses when products marketed as medical foods do not do what they claim to do.

A number of publications by and for health care professionals express concern about unsupported claims for foods that purport to be medical foods. For example. a recent edition of a book published by the United States Pharmacopeial Convention, Inc., *USP DI, Volume I, Drug Information for the Health Core Professional* (Ref. 8), lists enteral nutrition products that are formulated to meet nutrient requirements for individuals with specific diseases but states: "In general, scientific evidence for efficacy of these products is weak and requires further study." The l990 LSRO/FASEB report "Guidelines for the Scientific Review of Enteral Food Products for Special Medical Purposes" (Ref. 1) noted that products containing substances such as essential amino acids, peptides. and medium-chain triglycerides were available and that such products were represented as being useful for the dietary management of diseases and disorders. However, the report also stated that clinical trials of these preparations were limited, and that "none has fully confirmed or refuted the putative advantages of these products over ordinary nutritionally adequate preparations."

III. Clarification of the Medical Food Definition

In the preamble to one of the proposed rules implementing the 1990 amendments, FDA advised that it considered the statutory medical food definition to narrowly constrain the types of products that can be considered to be medical foods (56 FR 60366 at 60377). As noted previously in this document, however, the agency recognizes that the universe of products that purport to be medical foods has expanded beyond the statutory definition of a medical food to include foods that are more appropriately foods for special dietary use. In part, this expansion has occurred because many have difficulty distinguishing between medical foods and foods for special dietary use. While the agency recognizes that some ambiguity exists in the distinction between these two types of foods, the statutory language provides several bases on which to distinguish medical foods from foods for special dietary use.

A. "Distinctive Nutritional Requirements"

A fundamental element of the medical food definition that distinguishes this type of product from a food for special dietary use is the statutory requirement that a medical food be intended to meet distinctive nutritional requirements of a disease or condition. Under 21 U.S.C. 360ee(b)(3), distinctive nutritional requirements must be based on recognized scientific principles and established by medical evaluation. The law does not define what constitutes a "distinctive nutritional requirement," however, and there is more than one possible interpretation. FDA welcomes public comment on what definition of "distinctive nutritional requirement" will best protect and promote the public health. The agency is suggesting two possible interpretations of this phase.

1. Physiological Interpretation of "Distinctive Nutritional Requirement"

"Distinctive nutritional requirement" may be interpreted to refer to the body's requirement for specific amounts of nutrients to maintain homeostasis (the state of equilibrium in the body with respect to various functions and to the chemical compositions of the fluids and tissues) and sustain life; that is, the amount of each nutrient that must be available for use in the metabolic and physiological processes necessary to sustain life.

The nutritional requirements of healthy people for specific nutrients reflect their quantitative and qualitative requirements for absorbed nutrients (i.e., the physiological requirement for the nutrient), with adjustments for common inefficiencies associated with absorption, metabolism, and retention. However, the dietary management of patients with specific diseases requires, in some instances, the ability to meet nutritional requirements that differ substantially from the needs of healthy persons. For example, in establishing the recommended dietary allowances for the general, healthy population, the Food and Nutrition Board of the Institute of Medicine, National Academy of Sciences recognized that different or distinctive physiologic requirements may exist for certain persons with "special nutritional needs arising from metabolic disorders, chronic diseases, injuries, premature birth, other medical conditions, and drug therapies" (Ref. 9), Thus, the distinctive nutritional needs associated with a disease reflect the total amount needed by a healthy person to support life or maintain homeostasis, adjusted for the distinctive changes in the nutritional needs of the patient as a result of the effects of the disease process on absorption, metabolism, and excretion. These distinctive nutritional requirements may be greater than, less than, or in a narrower range of tolerance than for an otherwise healthy individual.

Under this physiological interpretation of "distinctive nutritional requirements, "medical foods" are foods that are formulated to aid in the dietary management of a specific disease or health-related condition that causes distinctive nutritional requirements that are different from the nutritional requirements of healthy people. Foods for special dietary use, on the other hand, are foods that are specially formulated to meet a special dietary need, such as a food allergy or difficulty in swallowing, but that provide nutrients intended to meet ordinary nutritional requirements. The special dietary needs addressed by these foods do not reflect a nutritional problem per se; that is, the physiological requirements for nutrients necessary to maintain life or homeostasis addressed by foods for special dietary use are the same as those of normal, healthy persons. These foods are formulated in such a way that only the ingredients or physical form of the diet is different. For example, a person who has difficulty swallowing solid food may have a special dietary need for a food that is in liquid form, but this special dietary need does not change his or her physiologic nutrient requirements. Similarly, a person who is allergic to specific food proteins (e.g., gluten) may need foods specially formulated not to contain these proteins. However, the specially formulated food still would provide the same amount of protein (i.e., amino acids) as is needed by the general population because the quantitative and qualitative amount of protein required by the body is similar in both healthy and protein-sensitive patients. Thus, foods for special dietary use are foods that are intended to meet ordinary nutritional requirements through special dietary means.

2. Alternative Interpretation of "Distinctive Nutritional Requirement"

"Distinctive nutritional requirement" may also be interpreted to encompass physical or physiological limitations in a person's ability to ingest or digest conventional foods, as well as distinctive physiological nutrient requirements. The FASEB report on medical foods stated that medical foods are for "patients with limited or impaired capacity to ingest, digest, absorb, or metabolize ordinary foodstuffs or certain nutrients contained therein, or (who) have other special medically determined nutrient requirements" (Ref.1). This definition would include uses that a purely physiological definition of "distinctive nutritional requirements" would exclude, such as foods intended for persons not able to ingest foods in certain physical forms (e.g., solid food), foods intended for persons who need a concentrated form of nutrition because of reduced appetite as a result of disease or convalescence), or foods intended for persons who may have other physical limitations on the amount or composition of food that they can consume. Although these types of conditions do not necessarily result in nutrient needs different from those of healthy persons, they represent a situation where it may be necessary that the food be formulated and manufactured within very narrow tolerances to ensure that the food provides most or all of the essential nutrients, as the persons for whom the food is intended may not be able to eat a variety of foods to ensure that they meet their nutrient requirements.

Therefore, it may be appropriate to define "distinctive nutritional requirements" to include those requirements that result from a disease or condition that cause a physical or physiological limitation in the ability of a person to ingest or digest conventional nutrient sources and result in that person needing specially formulated foods to meet part or all of their daily nutrient needs. Defining this term in this way may be appropriate because these circumstances create nutritional needs that are more narrowly defined than those of healthy persons, because the patient is relying on only a limited number of foods or a single food for sustenance. The agency asks for comments on whether persons with an impaired ability to ingest or digest specific foods because of a disease or condition, or who have physical or physiological limitations that cause them to rely on an enteral nutrition product for a significant part or all of their nutrient needs, have "distinctive nutritional requirements" within the meaning or the medical food definition.

B. "Under the Supervision of a Physician"

The second element of the medical food definition that distinguishes a medical food from a food for special dietary use is the statutory requirement that a medical food be "formulated to be consumed or administered enterally under the supervision of a physician." As stated in the preamble to the proposed rule implementing the nutrition labeling requirements of the 1990 amendments (56 FR 60366 at 60377), "under the supervision of a physician" means that the intended use of a medical food is for the dietary management of a patient receiving active and ongoing medical supervision (e.g., in a health care facility or as an outpatient). The physician determines that the medical food is necessary to the patient's overall medical care, and the patient consults the physician on a recurring basis.

Medical foods are intended for the dietary management of patients who have a short-term or long-term medical need for a particular nutrient or combination of nutrients to meet distinctive nutritional requirements. The use of a medical food requires ongoing physician oversight to ensure that the food effectively meets the distinctive nutritional requirements of the patient's disease or condition, and that the use of an enteral medical food is the appropriate means (i.e., as opposed to a patient requiring a parenteral nutrition product) to meet the patient's distinctive nutritional requirements. Therefore, medical foods are foods that are an integral components of the clinical management of a patient. Medical foods are not foods simply recommended by a physician as part of an overall diet designed to reduce the risk of a disease or medical condition, to lose or maintain weight, or to ensure the consumption of a healthy diet. Foods recommended by a physician for these purposes may be foods for special dietary use, but they are not medical foods.

C. "Specific Dietary Management"

The third fundamental element of the definition of a medical food that distinguishes a medical food from a food for special dietary use is the statutory requirement that a medical food be intended for the specific dietary management of a disease or condition. The term "specific dietary management" in the statutory definition of medical foods evidences that Congress intended these foods to be an integral part of the clinical treatment of patients. Consistent with this interpretation of this term, the LSRO/ FASEB Panel concluded that the objectives of incorporating the use of medical foods into patient management were, in part, to "ameliorate clinical manifestations of the disease," "favorably influence the disease process," and "positively influence morbidity and mortality (patient

outcomes)" (Ref. 1). There is no language corresponding to "specific dietary management" in the statutory definition applicable to foods for special dietary use. Thus, although they may be useful in supplying the special dietary needs of patients who have a disease or
other condition that prevents them from eating normally, foods for special dietary use, unlike medical foods, are not specifically tailored for use as the nutritional component of the patient's treatment.

D. Summary

The statutory definitions of medical foods and foods for special dietary use overlap to the extent that both categories encompass foods that are intended for use by sick people. The differences in the statutory definitions evidence, however, that Congress intended foods for special dietary use under section 411(c)(3)(A) of the act to be a broader category of foods for use by people with special dietary needs or desires, while it intended medical foods to be a narrower category of foods for use by people with particular diseases or conditions that have distinctive nutritional requirements. Since a medical food must address the "distinctive nutritional requirements" of a disease or condition, a medical food is suitable only for use by patients with that disease or condition. Of course, it is possible for more than one disease or condition to create the same distinctive nutritional requirements. A product that is intended to address the distinctive nutritional requirements of a particular disease is a medical food, even though some of those requirements may also be created by other diseases. A product that is designed to address a problem that is common to several diseases, but not the full range of requirements of any specific disease, would be a food for special dietary use; For example, the distinctive nutritional requirements of burn patients include a greater energy requirement due to hypermetabolism and a requirement for dietary glutamine because endogenous synthesis of this amino acid does not meet the metabolic requirement. Thus, a product formulated to meet the higher energy requirement due to the hypermetabolic state, but which does not meet the requirement for glutamine, would be a food for special dietary use and not a medical food because it does not meet the full range of distinctive nutritional requirements in patients with burn injuries.

IV. Need for Substantiation of Nutritional Efficacy and Claims Made in Product Labeling

Because of their intended use in supplying the distinctive nutritional needs of patients who are ill or otherwise medically vulnerable, it is essential that medical foods be appropriately formulated for the particular disease or condition for which they are labeled. Moreover, because the statutory definition of a medical food provides that these foods are part of the clinical management of a disease or condition, the definition necessarily incorporates a requirement that the product actually meet the distinctive nutritional requirements for the disease or condition. It is not enough that a manufacturer merely declare or subjectively intend that the product be used for the dietary management of patients with certain diseases or conditions. If the product, as formulated and consumed, does not actually meet those distinctive requirements, it would violate the act. Under any other view, the medical foods category would merely create a safe harbor for fraudulent claims targeted at those who are most vulnerable.

Other elements of the statutory definition support this view. In defining the term "medical food" in the Orphan Drug Amendments, Congress included the requirement that distinctive nutritional requirements of a disease or condition exist, and that they be based on recognized scientific principles and established by medical evaluation. Thus, Congress established a strict standard for when a food qualifies as a medical food. The establishment of this strict standard for distinctive nutritional requirements necessarily implies an expectation that this standard will in fact be met.

Acceptance of the manufacturer's intent that the product meets the special needs of the disease, without objective information to support the manufacturer's intent, would establish a subjective standard that would provide no assurance that the statutory standard has been met. Moreover, such a standard would ignore the fundamental differences between a medical food and other types of food. As stated above, a medical food is intended for use as the source of nutrients that are necessary in the medical management of a particular disease or condition. Thus, it is crucial to the health of the patient. No other type of food, including food for special dietary use, has such a direct relationship to the health of an individual. It is therefore necessary that the physician be able to rely on the medical food to effectively meet the distinctive nutritional requirements of the patient.

Finally, the statutory scheme for regulation of claims relating to health and disease confirms the appropriateness of a strong standard for substantiation of the nutritional efficacy of medical foods. The act establishes a range of circumstances under which claims relating to health and disease may be made. At one end of the spectrum are conventional foods, which under section 403(r) of the act may bear a health claim only if FDA determines:

based on the totality of publicly available scientific evidence (including evidence from well-designed studies conducted in a manner which is consistent with generally recognized scientific procedures and principles) that there is significant scientific agreement, among experts qualified by scientific training and experience to evaluate such claims, that the claim is supported by such evidence

At the other end of the spectrum are drugs, whose effectiveness in -diagnosing, curing, mitigating, treating, or preventing disease must be established by substantial evidence, defined as:

evidence consisting of adequate and well-controlled investigations, including clinical investigations, by experts qualified by scientific training and experience to evaluate the effectiveness of the drug involved, on the basis of which it could fairly and responsibly be concluded by such experts that the drug will have the effect it purports or is represented to have under the conditions of use prescribed, recommended, or suggested in the labeling or proposed labeling thereof.
(Section 505(d)(7) of the act (21 U.S.C, 355(d)(7)).)

Clearly, medical foods fall somewhere between these two points, and the statutory scheme therefore requires some level of substantiation for a medical food's claimed usefulness in the dietary management of disease.

When Congress enacted authorization for health claims on conventional foods, it provided that such claims would be permitted only if FDA determined that the substance-disease relationship that is the subject of the claim is supported by significant scientific agreement among experts, The House Report for the 1990 Amendments states: "The standard is intended to be a strong one. The bill requires that the Secretary have a high level of confidence that the claim is valid" (Ref, 10). The establishment of a"strong" scientific standard was necessary to ensure that claims were supported by adequate scientific evidence so that they would not be misleading, and so that consumers could have confidence in the scientific validity of the claimed substance-disease relationship. Thus, even a health claim for a food intended to be used by healthy individuals must meet a high standard.

The reasons for requiring a strong standard of substantiation apply with even more force to medical foods. The statutory definition of a medical food states that such a food must be intended for the specific dietary management of a disease or condition for which distinctive nutritional requirements, based on recognized scientific principles, are established by medical evaluation. As discussed earlier, this aspect of the definition makes it clear that Congress intended that claims made for medical foods be supported by scientific evidence, and it also constitutes a scientific standard that must be met for a food to be a medical food. The nature of these products (i.e., their intended use in the nutritional management of people affected by a disease or other condition) and the exemptions (i.e., from health claim requirements applicable to conventional foods) provided for them by virtue of their status as medical foods necessitate at least as much substantiation to support claims made for medical foods as for health claims on conventional foods. It would make no sense to establish a standard for claims on medical foods that was lower than the standard for health claims that are made for foods sold to healthy people.

The agency is concerned that many claims made for products marketed as medical foods are not supported by adequate scientific evidence, and that these unsupported claims result in the inappropriate use of some products by patients and physicians when effective alternative nutritional strategies for managing the disease are available. One medical expert on enteral nutrition formulas voiced this concern by stating that since the:

> introduction of nutritional support * * * as a specific therapeutic entity in the 1960's, a number of claims have been made, and widely believed, regarding its ability to improve the natural history of many diseases. However, these claims have been disseminated in the absence of supportive data from prospective randomized controlled trials * * *; in fact, when such studies have been performed. they have by and large not been able to demonstrate that [nutritional support] does improve morbidity and/or mortality.

(Ref.11)

A physician relies on the claims made for medical foods on their labels and in their labeling as a significant factor in deciding whether to use a particular medical food in the clinical management of a patient. Thus, it is essential that the claims made for such a product present an accurate interpretation of the scientific evidence concerning the usefulness of that product or specific formulation. It is critical for the safe and appropriate use of the medical food that the claims made for it are accurate and unbiased, and that they are based on a critical evaluation of the science available to the manufacturer. The need for physicians and patients to have confidence that any claim that a product is a medical food formulated for the specific dietary management of a disease or condition requires that a strong standard of substantiation be in place. A strong standard of substantiation would be one that requires that all pertinent data be considered in the formulation of the product and in the development of any claims about its use.

Further, the misbranding provisions of the act do not permit a food, including a medical food, to bear misleading labeling claims (section 403(a) of the act). Claims may be misleading not only because of affirmative representations made in the labeling, but also because the labeling fails to reveal facts material in the light of such representations with respect to consequences which may result from the use of the food under the conditions of use prescribed in the labeling or under usual or customary conditions of use (section 201(n) of the act). Thus, a medical food that bears claims that are not based on all the information available, and that do not permit the consumer or physician to make an informed choice, may be misbranded.

In summary, the intended uses of medical foods, the statutory definition of a medical food, and the statutory scheme for regulating health and disease claims all point to the need for a strong standard of scientific evidence for the composition and effectiveness of medical foods to provide assurance to health care providers and patients of the nutritional utility of these products. The standard should be no less demanding than for health claims for foods intended for the healthy general population. Moreover, because medical foods are intended for use in the clinical management of seriously ill and injured patients, it may be appropriate and necessary to apply a more stringent standard to the scientific evidence used to support claims made for medical foods. The agency's preliminary view is that the scientific standard contained in the statutory medical food definition may require some of the same types of data for medical foods as are needed to support drug claims (e.g., data from clinical investigations). The agency asks for comments regarding how stringent a scientific standard is necessary to ensure the safe and appropriate use of a medical food for a particular disease or condition.

V. Agency Plans

The agency is soliciting comments to initiate a reevaluation of its approach to the regulation of the broad group of heterogenous products marketed as medical foods and whether this approach serves the best interests of the consumers of such products. If the current regulatory approach is not adequate, the agency is interested in how it can improve the regulatory regime for medical foods to best serve those interests. FDA will review and consider all comments received. While this reevaluation is ongoing, however, the agency advises that it intends to continue to take regulatory action when necessary to protect consumers from unsafe or fraudulent products marketed as medical foods.

VI. Economic Issues

Under Executive Order 12866, FDA will be required to consider the costs and benefits of any proposed regulations pertaining to medical foods when regulations are proposed. In addition, under the Regulatory Flexibility Act and the Small Business Regulatory Enforcement and Fairness Act, FDA will be required to consider the impacts on small entities of any such regulations.

The primary benefit of any proposed change in the requirements applicable to medical foods will be a reduction in the health risks posed by medical foods that meet existing requirements. In addition, changes in the requirements applicable to medical foods that specify the level of scientific support required to make claims concerning the product will mean that consumers will have assurance that the claims are valid, and that the claims that are made provide reliable information. Other benefits will derive from the elimination of fraudulent and unsupported claims which will save consumers and third-party payers money and will improve patient health because people will use products that are appropriate for their conditions instead of relying on those bearing unsupported claims that do not have a positive impact on their conditions.

FDA asks for comments and information on the current health risks posed by medical foods meeting existing CGMP, labeling, and other applicable regulations. FDA also asks for comments on the degree to which these health risks may be reduced by additional regulation of medical foods, such as quality control requirements and additional CGMP and labeling regulations.

The primary cost of any proposed change will be the difference between the current cost of producing and marketing medical foods and the anticipated cost of producing and marketing medical foods under the proposed change. For example. relevant costs may include the cost of changing labels, generating particular types of information for labels, changing production methods or facilities to accommodate new CGMP requirements, the generation of additional information to establish product safety and effectiveness. and the cost of any uncertainty or delays associated with a potential pre market notification process.

FDA asks for comments on the costs that would be generated if medical foods were subject to additional regulatory requirements, such as quality control requirements, specific CGMP requirements. and labeling regulations. FDA also asks for comments on the impacts on small entities that would result if medical foods were subject to additional regulatory requirements of the type discussed in this document.

VII. Summary

Patients rely on medical foods to meet the distinctive nutritional needs resulting from their disease or condition, and, therefore, medical foods are often a significant part of the clinical management of these patients. Despite the importance of medical foods, however, existing regulations do not provide clear guidance on what products should be considered to be medical foods or on requirements to ensure that these foods do what they purport to do and are safe for their intended use. There is no regulatory framework that establishes specific quality assurance requirements. ensures the safety of medical foods under their intended conditions of use, ensures that they provide the nutrients that they claim to provide within safe ranges, or ensures that the benefits claimed for their purported use are supported by adequate scientific evidence. Therefore, the agency asks for comments on the following questions:

1. Is FDA's current approach to the regulation of medical foods adequate to ensure that food products claimed to be medical foods are safe and that the claims that they bear are valid? Is there a need for FDA to change its approach to the regulation of medical foods to better serve the needs of the patient populations that consume such products, and if so, what should the regulatory regime for medical foods be?

2. What factors should FDA consider applying as criteria to determine what products meet the statutory definition of a medical food? Should the agency apply a physiological interpretation of "distinctive nutritional requirements" in determining whether a product is a medical food, or should medical foods also include products that are used for patients with ingestion or digestion problems but with otherwise "normal" nutrient requirements? Would the latter interpretation be consistent with the act?

3. What requirements are necessary to ensure the safe and appropriate use of:(a) Products that meet the statutory definition of a medical food? (b) products that have been marketed as medical foods but that do not meet the statutory definition of a medical food?

Examples might include requirements that address product composition, current good manufacturing practice and quality control procedures, labeling requirements, and standards governing claims about the product and for foods that may be used as a sole item of the diet.

4. To ensure the safety and effectiveness of a medical food, should the agency require that the manufacturer notify FDA before marketing the product, and that it submit evidence that establishes that the product will be safe for its intended use and that any claims made for the product are supported by sound science? What information should be included in such a submission?

5. What standard should be used to determine the safety of a medical food?

6. What quantity and quality of scientific evidence should be required to establish that a disease or condition has distinctive nutritional requirements based on recognized scientific principles?

7. What quantity and quality of scientific evidence should be required to support the validity of claims made for medical foods?

8. What information should be included on the label of a medical food or otherwise disclosed to health care professionals and consumers? Should the amount and detail of the information to be disclosed depend on the types of claims made for the medical food or on other characteristics of the product? What methods would be most effective in communicating information on the intended uses, benefits, and other characteristics of a medical food to enable physicians and consumers to make informed decisions regarding its use (e.g., labels, package inserts, detailed summaries of the science upon which a firm is basing the claims made for its product)?

9. Should the agency develop regulations specifying quality control standards and procedures and current good manufacturing practice requirements for medical foods? What types of requirements are necessary (e.g., expiration dating, analysis of nutrient content, microbiological safety measurements, etc.)?

10. How should FDA monitor the safety and effectiveness of medical foods already on the market? What elements are necessary components of an effective postmarket surveillance system for these products? Should a postmarket surveillance system for medical foods include requirements and procedures for the collection and reporting to FDA of safety- and efficacy-related product defects adverse reaction reports, and complaints by health care professionals and consumers? Should manufacturers be required to collect information describing the outcomes associated with the use of medical food products in designated patient categories that would be available to FDA, health care providers, and consumers?

VIII. Comments

Interested persons may, on or before February 27, 1997, submit to the Dockets Management Branch (address above) written comments regarding this proposal. Two copies of any comments are to be submitted, except that individuals may submit one copy. Comments are to be identified with the docket number found in brackets in the heading of this document. Received comments may be seen in the office above between 9a.m. and 4 p.m., Monday through Friday.

IX. References

The following references have been placed on display in the Dockets Management Branch (address above) and may be seen by interested persons between 9 a.m. and 4 p.m., Monday through Friday.

1. Talbot, J. M., "Guidelines for the Scientific Review of Enteral Food Products for Special Medical Purposes," prepared for the Food and Drug Administration under FDA Contract No. 223-88-2124 by the Life Sciences Research Office, Federation of American Societies for Experimental Biology, Bethesda, MD, 1990.

2.Fisher, K. D., J. M. Talbot, and C. I.Carr, "A Review of Foods for Medical Purposes: Specially Formulated Products for Nutritional Management of Medical Conditions," prepared for the Food and Drug Administration under Contract No. FDA 223-75-2090 by the Life Sciences Research Office. Federation of American Societies for Experimental Biology, Bethesda. MD, 1977.

3. Hattan. D.G., and D. R.Mackey. "A Review of Medical Foods: Enterally Administered Formulations Used in the Treatment of Diseases and Disorders," *Food Drug Cosmetic Law Journal, 44:479-502*1989.

4. Health Hazard Evaluation No.1470, Food and Drug Administration Center for Food Safety and Applied Nutrition, 200 C St. SW., Washington. DC. April 25.1986.

5. FDA Enforcement Report, August 23, 1989, Rockville, MD.

6. FDA Enforcement Report. May 19,1993, Rockville, MD.

7. FDA Enforcement Report. July 28, 1993. Rockville, MD.

8. The United States Pharmacopeial Convention, Inc.,*USP DI, Drug Information for the Health Gore Professional, Volume I,* Rand McNally, Taunton, MS, 1996.

9. Subcommittee on the Tenth Edition of the RDA's, Food and Nutrition Board, Commission on Life Sciences, National Research Council, "Recommended Dietary Allowances, 10th ed.," National Academy Press, Washington, DC, 1989.

10. H. Rept. 101-538,101stCong., 2d sess., 19, "Nutrition Labeling and Education Act of 1990," June 13, 1990.

11. Koretz, R. L.. *A Critical Look at the Trials.* Symposium #2, Immunonutrition in the ICU, In: Proceedings of the 19th Clinical Congress, American Society forParenteral andEnteral Nutrition, Miami, FL, pp.97-103, 1995.

This document is issued under sections 4, 5, and 6 of the Fair Packaging and Labeling Act (15 U.S.C: 1453,1454, 1455); sections 201,301, 402,403, 404, 405, 409,411, 412,501, 502, 503, 505, and 701 of the Federal Food, Drug, and Cosmetic Act (21 U.S.C. 321, 331, 342, 343,344, 345, 348, 350, 350a, 351,352, 353, 355,371); and 21 U.S.C. 360ee(b)(3) (section 5(b)(3) of the Orphan Drug Amendments of 1988, as amended by Pub. L. 100-290).

Dated: October 31, 1996.

William B. Schultz,
Deputy Commissioner for Policy.

[FR Doc. 96-30441 Filed 11-27-96; 8:45 am]

BILLING CODE 4160-01-P

APPENDIX II Advance Notice of Proposed Rulemaking Extension of Comment Period

DEPARTMENT OF HEALTH AND HUMAN SERVICES

Food and Drug Administration

21 CFR Ch.I.

[Docket No. 96N-0364]

RIN 0910-AA20

Regulation of Medical Foods; Extension of Comment Period

AGENCY: Food and Drug Administration

Action: Advance notice of proposed rulemaking; extension of comment period.

SUMMARY: The food and Drug Administration (FDA) is extending to April 28, 1997, the comment period for the advance notice of proposed rulemaking for the regulation of medical foods that published in the Federal Register of November 29, 1996. This action is being taken in response to several requests from interested persons for an extension of the comment period on this document.

DATES: Written comments by April 28, 1997.

ADDRESSES: Submit written comments to the Dockets Management Branch (MFA-305), Food and Drug Administration, 12420 Parklawn Dr., rm. 1-23, Rockville, MD 20857.

FOR FURTHER INFORMATION CONTACT: Robert J. Moore, Center for Food Safety and Applied Nutrition (HFS-456), Food and Drug Administration, 200 C St. SW., Washington, DC 20204, 202-205-4605.

SUPPLEMENTARY INFORMATION: In the Federal Register of November 29, 1996 (61 FR 606611, FDA published an advance notice of proposed rulemaking for the regulation of medical foods. Interested persons were given until February 27, 1997, to comment on the advance notice of proposed rulemaking.

FDA has received requests for an extension of the comment period from: Manufacturers, a trade organization representing manufacturers of medical foods, and a professional society representing health care providers and research scientists. The interested parties stated in their requests for an extension of the comment period that such an extension would help ensure that the agency receives comprehensive and carefully researched information from experts to consider in response to the notice. After careful consideration of the requests submitted to the agency, FDA has decided to grant an extension of the comment period until April 28, 1997.

Interested persons may, on or before April 28, 1997, submit to the Dockets Management Branch (address above) written comments regarding this advanced notice of proposed rulemaking. Two copies of any comments are to be submitted, except that individuals may submit one copy. Comments are to be identified with the docket number found in brackets in the heading of this document. Received comments may be seen in the office above between 9 a.m. and 4 p.m., Monday through Friday.

INDEX